# *I Can Make You Thin*
# 90-DAY
# SUCCESS
# JOURNAL

*Also by Paul McKenna*

INSTANT CONFIDENCE!

I CAN MAKE YOU THIN

CHANGE YOUR LIFE IN SEVEN DAYS

I CAN MEND YOUR BROKEN HEART
(with Hugh Willbourn)

# I Can Make You Thin
# 90-DAY
# SUCCESS
# JOURNAL

## PAUL McKENNA Ph.D.

Edited by Michael Neill

BANTAM PRESS

LONDON · TORONTO · SYDNEY · AUCKLAND · JOHANNESBURG

TRANSWORLD PUBLISHERS
61-63 Uxbridge Road, London W5 5SA
a division of The Random House Group Ltd

RANDOM HOUSE SOUTH AFRICA (PTY) LTD
Isle of Houghton, Corner of Boundary and Carse O'Gowrie Roads,
Houghton 2198, South Africa

Published 2006 by Bantam Press
a division of Transworld Publishers
Copyright © Paul McKenna 2006

The right of Paul McKenna to be identified
as the author of this work has been asserted in accordance
with sections 77 and 78 of the Copyright, Designs and
Patents Act 1988.

A catalogue record for this book is available
from the British Library.

ISBN 978 0593 050569 (from Jan 07)
ISBN 0593 050568

Printed in Great Britain by Scotprint, East Lothian

9 10 8

Papers used by Transworld Publishers are natural, recyclable products
made from wood grown in sustainable forests. The manufacturing processes
conform to the environmental regulations of the country of origin.

JAN 11, 2013

# Your Success Calendar

*Start date* Nov 5/09 *Finish date* _____

| ✓ | 2 | 3 | 4 | 5 | 6 | 7 | 8 | 9 | 10 |
|---|---|---|---|---|---|---|---|---|---|
| 11 | 12 | 13 | 14 | 15 | 16 | 17 | 18 | 19 | 20 |
| 21 | 22 | 23 | 24 | 25 | 26 | 27 | 28 | 29 | 30 |
| 31 | 32 | 33 | 34 | 35 | 36 | 37 | 38 | 39 | 40 |
| 41 | 42 | 43 | 44 | 45 | 46 | 47 | 48 | 49 | 50 |
| 51 | 52 | 53 | 54 | 55 | 56 | 57 | 58 | 59 | 60 |
| 61 | 62 | 63 | 64 | 65 | 66 | 67 | 68 | 69 | 70 |
| 71 | 72 | 73 | 74 | 75 | 76 | 77 | 78 | 79 | 80 |
| 81 | 82 | 83 | 84 | 85 | 86 | 87 | 88 | 89 | 90 |

*Cross each day off your success calendar as you work through the programme ...*

# A Welcome Letter from Paul McKenna, Ph.D.

**Dear Reader,**

I don't know whether you have picked up this 90-day success journal because of something you've seen on television, read in a newspaper or been told by a friend, or just because it caught your eye in a bookshop, but I want you to know that if you're ready to finally shed that weight and keep it off for life, you're in for a real treat!

I don't care if you have been overweight all your life, if you're a late-night snacker, binge-eater, or if your entire family is overweight – the research shows that if you follow my four golden rules to weight-loss success you will lose weight, as more than 70% of the people who have used this system over the past few years have found out to their delight. (By way of comparison, traditional weight-loss systems and diet programmes have on average only a 9% success rate.)

Having shared this system with over half a million people in the past year alone, I found that the one thing people kept asking for was a support tool – a way of keeping track of progress and keeping on track when old patterns once again began to rear their ugly heads.

Based on your feedback, I have now developed that support tool – a 90-day success journal, which will support and guide you over the next three months until you've firmly established the new habits of relating to food and your body that will last you for a lifetime.

> *'Keeping a journal will absolutely change your life in ways you've never imagined.'*
> OPRAH WINFREY

A recent study by Dr Ben Fletcher showed that when people change their routines they naturally lose weight, even though they aren't told to diet or exercise. To help you change your routine, I have packed this journal with simple, fun activities that will interrupt your old patterns of thinking and behaviour and help you to create and maintain new ones.

If you've never kept a journal before, prepare to be amazed at the difference it will make in your life. It's not just the act of writing things down or ticking boxes that focuses your thoughts and behaviours for success. It's the commitment you are making to yourself as you change your old routine and do something different that will disrupt the negative patterns and set you on a new course to a healthier way of eating and a happier way of life!

*To your success,*
**Paul McKenna**

# How to use this journal

The weight-loss system you are about to embark upon is the most successful in the world. If it were a pill I could sell it to a drug company for a billion dollars. But it's not a pill, it's a system – a system so simple that, at first, most people can't believe it will work for them.

The best thing is, you don't have to believe in it and there's no willpower required. All you have to do is just follow my instructions and your life will dramatically change for the better.

Here's how it all works ...

## Weekly themes

Each week, you will be introduced to a theme, ranging from understanding emotional eating to lightening up and having more fun in your life.

Most of these weekly themes relate to one of the key sections in *I Can Make You Thin* – if you haven't already got it, I highly recommend you pick up a copy both so you can do extra reading about the weekly themes and for the free CD (see point 7, opposite*) that will become a part of your daily routine.

# Daily thoughts and activities

On the left side of each daily entry, I will share with you one of my favourite quotes along with a simple thought or exercise you can do to solidify the changes you are making in how you think and act around food. On each facing page, you will find an eight-item 'Success Checklist'. These eight activities will be the keys to your success throughout this programme:

1   Eating when you are hungry
2   Eating what you *really* want
3   Eating consciously
4   Stopping when you are full
5   Drinking water
6   Moving your body
7   Listening to the mind-programming CD*
8   Doing the mirror exercise (from page 219)

It is important for you to know that while following the first four 'golden rules' is at the heart of my system, it is not necessary for you to do every single thing on every single day in order to succeed. In fact, I would be amazed if you did. This programme is about progress, not per-fection – and as long as you are doing most things on most days, you will make tangible progress towards your goals.

Underneath the success checklist, I've made space for you to make notes about one positive thing you've noticed today and at least one thing you're looking forward to tomorrow. Don't underestimate the power of these two simple observations. What you focus on in life expands, and by focusing on your positive experiences and positive expectancies, you will find yourself drawing more and more of what you want into your life.

## 'Review and renew' days

Every seventh day is set aside for review and renewal. This will give you a chance to reflect back on the week just gone and look forward to the week ahead. There are five things to record on your review days:

1   The best things that happened
2   The most challenging things that happened
3   Any new behaviours
4   What you learned
5   Your top priorities for the week ahead

You can see a sample 'Review and renew' day all filled in at the end of this section.

## Check-in days

Spread throughout the journal you will find six 'check-in' days. These are the only days I want you to weigh yourself during the programme. This is actually the one part of the journal you may skip altogether – looking great and feeling wonderful will always be a better measure of your progress than the numbers on a scale.

## One last thing before you begin ...

On check-in days, you will have the opportunity to read testimonials from people who have successfully used my system to lose weight and free up their bodies and minds from the patterns of obsessive dieting, emotional eating and faulty programming that kept them from living happily and at their desired weight.

The final testimonial in the book will be ... yours!

In order to prepare yourself to be truly amazed at how well you do on this programme, I want you to take a picture of yourself as you look now and paste or tape it into the 'Before' box on day 90. Don't worry if you hate being photographed or think you look terrible. By the time you've finished this programme, this will be your favourite picture in the world – a reminder of how things used to be and how far you've come in such a relatively short period of time.

If you've decided to weigh yourself on the check-in days, step on the scales now and write in your weight in the space underneath the picture. Be sure to fill in today's date as well. As soon as you've done these three things, you are ready to begin the transformation of a lifetime ...

# Sample Journal Entry

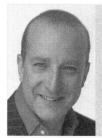

# DAY 59

## Review and renew

*'Reflect upon your present blessings, of which every man has many; not upon your past misfortunes, of which all men have some.'*

CHARLES DICKENS

Did you enjoy your week of eating mindfully? It doesn't have to end today – as you move into the final month of our time together, mindfulness can be a powerful ally as you continue to reprogramme your mind and body to be naturally thin. Take some time today to ask and answer these questions …

**1** The best things that happened this week were:

*Followed the rules 5 of 6 days; great meeting at work on Tuesday*

**2** My biggest challenges this week were:

*Binged on cake at party; the argument(!)*

**3** I did these things for the first time:

*Took the dogs for a walk because I actually wanted some exercise*

**4** What I learned was:

*One bad day doesn't have to ruin my week*

**5** My top three priorities for the week ahead are:

**a** *Drink more water*

**b** *Prepare sales reports for work*

**c** *Spend more time doing the mirror exercise*

# TODAY'S SUCCESS CHECKLIST

| | TICK | COMMENTS |
|---|---|---|
| **1** I ate when I was hungry | ✔ | |
| **2** I ate what I *really* wanted | ✔ | |
| **3** I ate consciously | ✔ | |
| **4** I stopped when full | ✔ | *Yaaay!* |
| **5** I drank water | ✔ | |
| **6** I moved my body | ☐ | |
| **7** I listened to the CD | ☐ | *Load CD into iPod* |
| **8** I did the mirror exercise | ✔ | |

## ONE **POSITIVE THING** I NOTICED TODAY...

*I think this really is working - I didn't even notice the*

*doughnuts had been and gone at work until the end of*

*the day*

## WHAT I'M **LOOKING FORWARD TO** TOMORROW...

*Meeting Brian for drinks down the pub*

# Week 1

# Starting Strong!

*'The greatest thing in this world
is not so much where we stand
as in what direction we are moving.'*

JOHANN WOLFGANG VON GOETHE

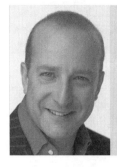

# DAY 1

## Begin with the end in mind

*'Start by doing what's necessary; then do what's possible; and suddenly you are doing the impossible.'*

ST FRANCIS OF ASSISI

Today, it begins – the first day of what will probably be an entirely new relationship with food and an entirely new relationship with your body. But where will it all end?

Take a few moments to do the following:

Close your eyes and imagine that it's 90 days from today. If it helps, you can actually mark the date on a real or imaginary calendar. Now travel out into the future until you are looking at a future, slimmer, happier you. When you're ready, step into that future you until you're seeing what they see, hearing what they hear, and feeling the wonderful feelings in your brand new body.

The more you allow yourself to really enjoy this feeling, the easier it will be to return to this visualisation again and again throughout the 90 days – and every time you do, you are programming your mind for success!

# TODAY'S SUCCESS CHECKLIST

|  | TICK | COMMENTS |
|---|---|---|
| **1** I ate when I was hungry | ☑ | _Semi-hungry_ |
| **2** I ate what I _really_ wanted | ☑ | _yes_ |
| **3** I ate consciously | ☑ | _Sometime_ |
| **4** I stopped when full | ☑ | _Sort off_ |
| **5** I drank water | ☐ | _NO — Tea, coffee_ |
| **6** I moved my body | ☑ | _Yes_ |
| **7** I listened to the CD | ☑ | _yes_ |
| **8** I did the mirror exercise | ☐ | _NO_ |

## ONE **POSITIVE THING** I NOTICED TODAY...

_I'm starting to feel better. Stomach not bloated, feels strange_

## WHAT I'M **LOOKING FORWARD TO** TOMORROW...

_Having energy to complete goals gym, clean apt. Not feeling so tired. Be HAPPY_

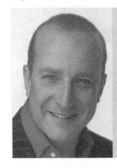

# DAY 2

## A picture of success

*'The human body is the best picture of the human soul.'*

LUDWIG WITTGENSTEIN

Have you ever seen one of those pictures of an athlete in the moment of victory? Even as we look at another person reaching their goal, our own resolve and will to win is strengthened.

Today, take some time to find a picture of something or someone that inspires you. Put it up somewhere where you'll see it every day (like the refrigerator!) or carry it around in your purse, wallet or even inside this journal. Whenever you need an extra dose of courage or determination, you can look at the picture and inspire yourself to success!

# TODAY'S SUCCESS CHECKLIST

| | TICK | COMMENTS |
|---|---|---|
| **1** I ate when I was hungry | ☑ | _Small amt_ |
| **2** I ate what I *really* wanted | ☑ | _Yes_ |
| **3** I ate consciously | ☑ | _Mostly_ |
| **4** I stopped when full | ☑ | _Yes_ |
| **5** I drank water | ☑ | |
| **6** I moved my body | ☑ | _Walked — Pac Dan Gar_ |
| **7** I listened to the CD | ☐ | _No_ |
| **8** I did the mirror exercise | ☐ | _No_ |

## ONE **POSITIVE THING** I NOTICED TODAY...

_(handwritten, illegible)_

## WHAT I'M **LOOKING FORWARD TO** TOMORROW...

_(handwritten, illegible)_

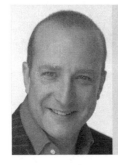

# DAY 3

## Empty your refrigerator

*'Part of the secret of success in life is to eat what you like
and let the food fight it out inside.'*

MARK TWAIN

You may have, in the past, been on one diet or another that
told you to empty your cupboards of any foods high in fat,
sugar, carbohydrates, or whatever food you were being
forbidden to eat.

My instructions for you are radically different:

Today, I want you to go to your refrigerator and
throw out any food that does not totally inspire you to
eat it. Chuck the diet soda. Throw out the low-fat
yogurts. Unless you love them, bin the sugar-free
popsicles. You'll know that you're done when there isn't
a single thing in your fridge that you wouldn't be
delighted to eat – and when you're next hungry, that's
exactly what I'm asking you to do!

# TODAY'S SUCCESS CHECKLIST

|  | TICK | COMMENTS |
|---|---|---|
| **1** I ate when I was hungry | ☑ | _CLOSE_ |
| **2** I ate what I *really* wanted | ☐ | |
| **3** I ate consciously | ☐ | |
| **4** I stopped when full | ☐ | |
| **5** I drank water | ☐ | |
| **6** I moved my body | ☐ | |
| **7** I listened to the CD | ☐ | |
| **8** I did the mirror exercise | ☐ | |

## ONE **POSITIVE THING** I NOTICED TODAY...

_[handwritten, illegible]_

## WHAT I'M **LOOKING FORWARD TO** TOMORROW...

_[handwritten, illegible]_

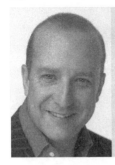

# DAY 4

## Accept yourself!

*'Everything in life that we really accept undergoes a change.'*
KATHERINE MANSFIELD

When we focus on our goals for the future, it can sometimes seem as though we are really rejecting who we are in the present.

Take a few minutes to stand in front of the mirror today and send love and approval to your body. Remember, acceptance doesn't mean that you don't want to change something – it just means that you are willing to accept that where you are now is where you are now.

# TODAY'S SUCCESS CHECKLIST

|  | TICK | COMMENTS |
|---|---|---|
| **1** I ate when I was hungry | ☐ | _____ |
| **2** I ate what I *really* wanted | ☐ | _____ |
| **3** I ate consciously | ☐ | _____ |
| **4** I stopped when full | ☐ | _____ |
| **5** I drank water | ☐ | _____ |
| **6** I moved my body | ☐ | _____ |
| **7** I listened to the CD | ☐ | _____ |
| **8** I did the mirror exercise | ☐ | _____ |

## ONE **POSITIVE THING** I NOTICED TODAY...

_____

_____

_____

## WHAT I'M **LOOKING FORWARD TO** TOMORROW...

_____

_____

_____

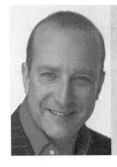

# DAY 5

## The best year of your life

*'You will think more than 50,000 thoughts today,
so you might as well make them big ones!'*

DONALD TRUMP

Chances are that if you're using this journal, you've already decided that it's time for a change. But you may not yet realize that you're probably thinking too small...

Close your eyes and vividly imagine it's a year from now and you have had your best year so far. What must have happened for that to be true?

Be specific about each area of your life: your health, your career, your relationships, your finances, your spirituality.

Remember it's very important to be clear. If you put vagueness out you will get vague results back. So take a few minutes and imagine your life has become outrageously better. Then, at least five times today, spend a few moments thinking about how good your life can be!

# TODAY'S SUCCESS CHECKLIST

| | TICK | COMMENTS |
|---|---|---|
| **1** I ate when I was hungry | ☐ | _____ |
| **2** I ate what I *really* wanted | ☐ | _____ |
| **3** I ate consciously | ☐ | _____ |
| **4** I stopped when full | ☐ | _____ |
| **5** I drank water | ☐ | _____ |
| **6** I moved my body | ☐ | _____ |
| **7** I listened to the CD | ☐ | _____ |
| **8** I did the mirror exercise | ☐ | _____ |

## ONE **POSITIVE THING** I NOTICED TODAY...

_____

_____

_____

## WHAT I'M **LOOKING FORWARD TO** TOMORROW...

_____

_____

_____

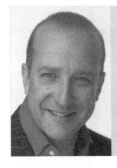

# DAY 6

## An attitude of gratitude

*'Feeling gratitude and not expressing it
is like wrapping a present and not giving it.'*
WILLIAM ARTHUR WARD

When we are wrapped up in our own worries and concerns, it is the easiest thing in the world to overlook all the good things we already have in our lives.

Today, we are going to reverse that pattern. Ask yourself to focus on what's already working well in your life. Ask and answer these questions each time you notice you are hungry. When you've fed your heart, it will be time to feed your body...

- Who do I love?
- Who loves me?
- What am I most grateful for in my life?
- What is it about that which makes me feel grateful?

# TODAY'S SUCCESS CHECKLIST

|  | TICK | COMMENTS |
|---|---|---|
| **1** I ate when I was hungry | ☐ | _____ |
| **2** I ate what I *really* wanted | ☐ | _____ |
| **3** I ate consciously | ☐ | _____ |
| **4** I stopped when full | ☐ | _____ |
| **5** I drank water | ☐ | _____ |
| **6** I moved my body | ☐ | _____ |
| **7** I listened to the CD | ☐ | _____ |
| **8** I did the mirror exercise | ☐ | _____ |

## ONE **POSITIVE THING** I NOTICED TODAY...

_____

_____

_____

## WHAT I'M **LOOKING FORWARD TO** TOMORROW...

_____

_____

_____

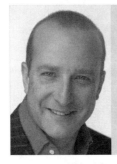

# DAY 7

## Review and renew

*'Hope is a renewable option: If you run out of it*
*at the end of the day, you get to start over in the morning.'*

BARBARA KINGSOLVER

Every seven days, I'm going to ask you to take time out to reflect on how far you've come and re-focus on where it is you are heading. Here's your very first chance to 'review and renew'…

**1** The best things that happened this week were:

**2** My biggest challenges this week were:

**3** I did these things for the first time:

**4** What I learned was:

**5** My top three priorities for the week ahead are:

a

b

c

# TODAY'S SUCCESS CHECKLIST

| | TICK | COMMENTS |
|---|---|---|
| **1** I ate when I was hungry | ☐ | _____ |
| **2** I ate what I *really* wanted | ☐ | _____ |
| **3** I ate consciously | ☐ | _____ |
| **4** I stopped when full | ☐ | _____ |
| **5** I drank water | ☐ | _____ |
| **6** I moved my body | ☐ | _____ |
| **7** I listened to the CD | ☐ | _____ |
| **8** I did the mirror exercise | ☐ | _____ |

## ONE **POSITIVE THING** I NOTICED TODAY...

_____

_____

_____

## WHAT I'M **LOOKING FORWARD TO** TOMORROW...

_____

_____

_____

# Week 2

# The Four
# Golden Rules

*'Simplicity is the ultimate sophistication.'*

Leonardo da Vinci

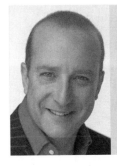

# DAY 8

## The four golden rules to losing weight forever

*'The main thing is to keep the main thing the main thing.'*
STEPHEN R. COVEY

This week, we'll go through each of the golden rules to success in a bit more depth and reinforce them as habits. For today, just imagine what it would be like to really eat this way …

Imagine yourself tuning into your body and noticing you're a little bit hungry. In the past, you might have ignored this sensation, but now you've learned to respect it. You ask your body what it wants and needs. To your amazement, it asks for a small bowl of pasta with a salad. (You were sure it was going to be chocolate cake and ice cream, weren't you?)

Resisting the urge to skip the pasta, you sit down for a wonderful, peaceful meal. Stopping to smell your food between each mouthful, you enjoy indulging in the sensation of the warm pasta melting in your mouth before sliding easily down your throat. Each bite of salad crunches in your mouth, and you can taste the water-rich juice from the lettuce and cucumber with every mouthful. Delicious!

Down towards the bottom of the bowl, you realize you are comfortably full. Imagine the sense of pride as you push away the rest of the bowl, knowing you are now in full control …

# TODAY'S SUCCESS CHECKLIST

| | TICK | COMMENTS |
|---|---|---|
| **1** I ate when I was hungry | ☐ | _____ |
| **2** I ate what I *really* wanted | ☐ | _____ |
| **3** I ate consciously | ☐ | _____ |
| **4** I stopped when full | ☐ | _____ |
| **5** I drank water | ☐ | _____ |
| **6** I moved my body | ☐ | _____ |
| **7** I listened to the CD | ☐ | _____ |
| **8** I did the mirror exercise | ☐ | _____ |

## ONE **POSITIVE THING** I NOTICED TODAY...

_____

_____

_____

## WHAT I'M **LOOKING FORWARD TO** TOMORROW...

_____

_____

_____

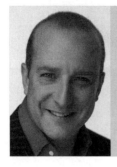

# DAY 9

## Rule 1: Eat when hungry

*'Once you learn to quit, it becomes a habit.'*

VINCENT LOMBARDI

I was amazed when someone told me that she was shocked to hear that one of the keys to losing weight and keeping it off was to eat when she was hungry.

'If I did that,' she told me, 'I'd never stop.'

Isn't it funny that some people are such experts on what they've never done?

It's time to end the self-inflicted torture and listen to your body instead!

Make this commitment:

*'I, _____, promise that for at least the next 81 days, I will eat whenever I'm hungry no matter how I feel about it.'*

# TODAY'S SUCCESS CHECKLIST

|  | TICK | COMMENTS |
|---|---|---|
| **1** I ate when I was hungry | ☐ | _____ |
| **2** I ate what I *really* wanted | ☐ | _____ |
| **3** I ate consciously | ☐ | _____ |
| **4** I stopped when full | ☐ | _____ |
| **5** I drank water | ☐ | _____ |
| **6** I moved my body | ☐ | _____ |
| **7** I listened to the CD | ☐ | _____ |
| **8** I did the mirror exercise | ☐ | _____ |

## ONE **POSITIVE THING** I NOTICED TODAY...

_____

_____

_____

## WHAT I'M **LOOKING FORWARD TO** TOMORROW...

_____

_____

_____

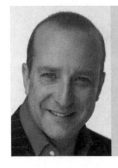

# DAY 10

## Rule 2: Eat what you really want, not what you think you should

*'The only way to get rid of a temptation is to yield to it.'*

OSCAR WILDE

There are NO forbidden foods in my system – you can eat anything you want any time you are hungry, providing you take the time to really, really enjoy eating it.

Fancy a bit of pasta?

Go for it.

Cake and ice cream calling to you?

As long as you're actually hungry, enjoy, enjoy, enjoy.

From this day forward, nothing is off-limits to you. Ever.

And if you still really want to say 'NO' to something, say it to the purveyors of sugar-free low-carb cardboard-tasting crap.

# TODAY'S SUCCESS CHECKLIST

|  | TICK | COMMENTS |
|---|---|---|

**1** I ate when I was hungry ☐ _____

**2** I ate what I *really* wanted ☐ _____

**3** I ate consciously ☐ _____

**4** I stopped when full ☐ _____

**5** I drank water ☐ _____

**6** I moved my body ☐ _____

**7** I listened to the CD ☐ _____

**8** I did the mirror exercise ☐ _____

## ONE **POSITIVE THING** I NOTICED TODAY...

_____

_____

_____

## WHAT I'M **LOOKING FORWARD TO** TOMORROW...

_____

_____

_____

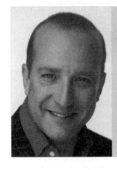

# DAY 11

## Rule 3: Eat consciously – enjoy each mouthful

*'Pleasure is the object, the duty and the goal of all rational creatures.'*

VOLTAIRE

Here's a little experiment for you to try today:

1 Create a 'sample platter' with a taste of each of your favourite foods – a bit of warm bread with butter, a slice of sharp cheddar cheese, a bite of a bar of chocolate, a bit of sushi, or anything that makes your mouth water just thinking about it.

2 When you've read through all these instructions, close your eyes and indulge your senses. Smell your food before eating it. See how long you can make each bite last. Most foods actually have more than one taste when you take the time to really savour them. In fact, if you really pay close attention, you will notice the tastes and textures changing as you chew them.

3 Notice which foods become more enjoyable the longer you take to eat them, and any which may become less enjoyable. Try and discover at least one new flavour in each food you sample.

Remember, the more you are willing to enjoy each mouthful, the thinner you are becoming!

# TODAY'S SUCCESS CHECKLIST

| | TICK | COMMENTS |
|---|---|---|
| **1** I ate when I was hungry | ☐ | _____ |
| **2** I ate what I *really* wanted | ☐ | _____ |
| **3** I ate consciously | ☐ | _____ |
| **4** I stopped when full | ☐ | _____ |
| **5** I drank water | ☐ | _____ |
| **6** I moved my body | ☐ | _____ |
| **7** I listened to the CD | ☐ | _____ |
| **8** I did the mirror exercise | ☐ | _____ |

## ONE **POSITIVE THING** I NOTICED TODAY...

_____

_____

_____

## WHAT I'M **LOOKING FORWARD TO** TOMORROW...

_____

_____

_____

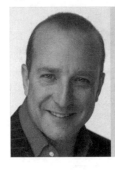

# DAY 12

## Rule 4: Stop when you think you're full

*'This life is not for complaint, but for satisfaction.'*

HENRY DAVID THOREAU

What's the first sign for you that your body is getting full and satisfied with what you've eaten?

Here are what some of the people on my seminars have said:

*I know I'm getting full when my stomach starts to grumble.*
*I know I'm getting full when the food stops tasting quite so good.*
*I know I'm getting full when I can't think of anything else I'd like to eat.*
*I know I'm getting full because I suspect I might be.*

What is it for you?

If you're not sure, take some time today to really tune in to your body as you eat and notice what the very first sign of satisfaction and fullness is for you. The more aware of your body's signals you become, the easier it will be for you to not only lose those extra pounds but to keep them off for good!

# TODAY'S SUCCESS CHECKLIST

| | TICK | COMMENTS |
|---|---|---|
| **1** I ate when I was hungry | ☐ | _____ |
| **2** I ate what I *really* wanted | ☐ | _____ |
| **3** I ate consciously | ☐ | _____ |
| **4** I stopped when full | ☐ | _____ |
| **5** I drank water | ☐ | _____ |
| **6** I moved my body | ☐ | _____ |
| **7** I listened to the CD | ☐ | _____ |
| **8** I did the mirror exercise | ☐ | _____ |

## ONE **POSITIVE THING** I NOTICED TODAY...

_____

_____

_____

## WHAT I'M **LOOKING FORWARD TO** TOMORROW...

_____

_____

_____

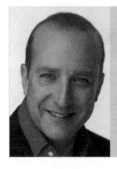

# DAY 13

## Revisiting the hunger scale

*'Living in balance and purity is the highest good
for you and the earth.'*

DEEPAK CHOPRA

Perhaps the most useful tool you can use in your quest for more pleasure and less weight is the hunger scale:

| **The Hunger Scale** |
| --- |
| 1 – Physically faint |
| 2 – Ravenous |
| 3 – Fairly hungry |
| 4 – Slightly hungry |
| 5 – Neutral |
| 6 – Pleasantly satisfied |
| 7 – Full |
| 8 – Stuffed |
| 9 – Bloated |
| 10 – Nauseous |

Remember, you ideally want to begin eating between 3 and 4 and finish eating around 6. The more you go to one extreme, the more likely you are to go to the other. By avoiding both extremes, you will be living your life in balance!

# TODAY'S SUCCESS CHECKLIST

|  | TICK | COMMENTS |
|---|---|---|
| **1** I ate when I was hungry | ☐ | _____ |
| **2** I ate what I *really* wanted | ☐ | _____ |
| **3** I ate consciously | ☐ | _____ |
| **4** I stopped when full | ☐ | _____ |
| **5** I drank water | ☐ | _____ |
| **6** I moved my body | ☐ | _____ |
| **7** I listened to the CD | ☐ | _____ |
| **8** I did the mirror exercise | ☐ | _____ |

## ONE **POSITIVE THING** I NOTICED TODAY...

_____

_____

_____

## WHAT I'M **LOOKING FORWARD TO** TOMORROW...

_____

_____

_____

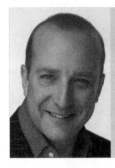

# DAY 14

## Review and renew

*'The more you praise and celebrate your life, the more there is in life to celebrate.'*

OPRAH WINFREY

You're two weeks into a brand new way of eating – how does it feel? Exciting? Scary? Both?

Prepare for tomorrow today by taking some time to review and renew ...

**1** The best things that happened this week were:

**2** My biggest challenges this week were:

**3** I did these things for the first time:

**4** What I learned was:

**5** My top three priorities for the week ahead are:

   **a**

   **b**

   **c**

# TODAY'S SUCCESS CHECKLIST

| | TICK | COMMENTS |
|---|---|---|
| **1** I ate when I was hungry | ☐ | _____ |
| **2** I ate what I _really_ wanted | ☐ | _____ |
| **3** I ate consciously | ☐ | _____ |
| **4** I stopped when full | ☐ | _____ |
| **5** I drank water | ☐ | _____ |
| **6** I moved my body | ☐ | _____ |
| **7** I listened to the CD | ☐ | _____ |
| **8** I did the mirror exercise | ☐ | _____ |

## ONE **POSITIVE THING** I NOTICED TODAY...

_____

_____

_____

## WHAT I'M **LOOKING FORWARD TO** TOMORROW...

_____

_____

_____

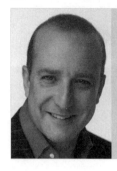

# DAY 15

## Your first check-in ...

*'You have to eat regularly to maintain your energy levels – if you starve your body, it simply stores everything that you do eat.'*

CINDY CRAWFORD

Congratulations! For two weeks now, you have been interrupting your old patterns of diet and exercise and building the foundations for a whole new way of relating to food, your emotions and your body. By the time you are finished with this journal, it will be as difficult for you to go back to your old way of doing things as it will be easy and natural to eat and live in a way that truly works for you.

Remember, this journal is designed to support you in creating the habits of empowered eating. Take a moment now to jot down anything you've already noticed about how things are changing ...

_____

_____

_____

_____

# Manjit Sahota **LOST 11 STONE**

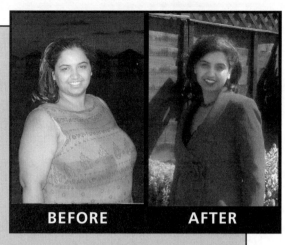

I have always been overweight and from early childhood been on every possible diet you could think of. After seeing my honeymoon pictures, I was distraught. That same week I saw Paul's book and started reading it at once. For a week, I followed the instructions and listened to the CD.

Something just clicked. I made losing weight into an objective and my mind was set. I've never been able to lose so much weight so easily before … and enjoy everything I was doing to achieve it!

I cannot overemphasize the value of the tools and techniques – and I can say that I had fun reading the book and that it made my dreams come true. I continue to use the tools and technique in other aspects of my life, too, with many positive outcomes.

I can simply say that it does what it says on the packet – these techniques changed my life and I made my dreams into reality.

## TODAY I WEIGH

# Week 3

# On the Sunny Side of the Street!

*'Things turn out best for the people who make the best of the way things turn out.'*

JOHN WOODEN

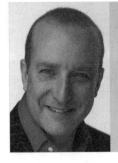

# DAY 16

## Accentuate the positive

*'The secret of staying young is to live honestly,
eat slowly, and lie about your age.'*

LUCILLE BALL

One of my favourite exercises we do on our NLP trainings
is called 'On the Sunny Side of the Street'. In groups of five
or six people, someone calls out something that would gen-
erally be thought of as negative. Everyone in the group then
has to come up with a way in which that could be perceived
as a positive. For example, if somebody said, 'I think about
food all the time', people in the group might respond:

'You must be an expert by now – maybe you could host
a talk show!'

'Wow – I bet that means you're a very sensual person!'

'At least you can think!'

The purpose of the exercise is not to convince yourself to
be happy about something you're not, but rather to recognize and increase your capacity to find the positive in the
midst of a challenge. Have a go right now …

1 Think of something you're a little bit unhappy about in
your life.

2 Come up with at least three ways it could be seen as a
good thing – the more outrageous the better!

# TODAY'S SUCCESS CHECKLIST

| | TICK | COMMENTS |
|---|---|---|
| **1** I ate when I was hungry | ☐ | _____ |
| **2** I ate what I *really* wanted | ☐ | _____ |
| **3** I ate consciously | ☐ | _____ |
| **4** I stopped when full | ☐ | _____ |
| **5** I drank water | ☐ | _____ |
| **6** I moved my body | ☐ | _____ |
| **7** I listened to the CD | ☐ | _____ |
| **8** I did the mirror exercise | ☐ | _____ |

## ONE **POSITIVE THING** I NOTICED TODAY...

_____

_____

_____

## WHAT I'M **LOOKING FORWARD TO** TOMORROW...

_____

_____

_____

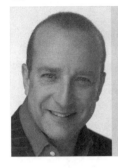

# DAY 17

## Eliminate the negative

*'Better to light a candle than to curse the darkness.'*

CHINESE PROVERB

Over the years, I have worked with any number of struggling actors and musicians who resented the rich and famous while simultaneously striving to join their ranks.

The problem with that is simple:

**It's difficult to become something if you hate it.**

Your unconscious mind craves consistency – and if you keep telling it that you hate all naturally thin people, it will do whatever it can to not let you become one of them.

There is something miraculously freeing about celebrating the success of others, even those people we don't particularly like. Try it as an experiment for the next few days. Whenever you hear about someone doing well, think something congratulatory. Bless their success instead of cursing it. Shortly this will become a new habit and you will become a more positive person.

And as you begin to wish the best for those who are thinner than you, your unconscious mind will begin to make you more like them!

# TODAY'S SUCCESS CHECKLIST

| | TICK | COMMENTS |
|---|---|---|
| **1** I ate when I was hungry | ☐ | _____ |
| **2** I ate what I *really* wanted | ☐ | _____ |
| **3** I ate consciously | ☐ | _____ |
| **4** I stopped when full | ☐ | _____ |
| **5** I drank water | ☐ | _____ |
| **6** I moved my body | ☐ | _____ |
| **7** I listened to the CD | ☐ | _____ |
| **8** I did the mirror exercise | ☐ | _____ |

## ONE **POSITIVE THING** I NOTICED TODAY...

_____

_____

_____

## WHAT I'M **LOOKING FORWARD TO** TOMORROW...

_____

_____

_____

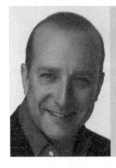

# DAY 18

## Approval, approval, approval, approval, approval

*'A man cannot be comfortable without his own approval.'*

MARK TWAIN

A lady came on one of my easy weight-loss seminars determined that this time things would be different. Whatever the programme was, she was going to follow it to the letter until she'd lost every pound she'd packed on since her last baby was born. But when I asked her to look in the mirror and approve of herself as she was, she wanted to leave the room.

'I've never approved of myself,' she confessed. 'I'm not sure I know how!'

Here is all that you need to do:

1 Begin by sending approval to your big toe, or any part of your body about which you are indifferent. Simply tell it that you approve of it and are willing to love it as it is right now.

2 Work your way through every part of your body until you can love and approve of EVERYTHING. If you've really never done this before, it's OK if it takes a few days or even weeks.

Remember, approval doesn't mean you won't change – it just means you won't be in terrible emotional pain while you do!

# TODAY'S SUCCESS CHECKLIST

|  | TICK | COMMENTS |
|---|---|---|
| **1** I ate when I was hungry | ☐ | _____ |
| **2** I ate what I *really* wanted | ☐ | _____ |
| **3** I ate consciously | ☐ | _____ |
| **4** I stopped when full | ☐ | _____ |
| **5** I drank water | ☐ | _____ |
| **6** I moved my body | ☐ | _____ |
| **7** I listened to the CD | ☐ | _____ |
| **8** I did the mirror exercise | ☐ | _____ |

## ONE **POSITIVE THING** I NOTICED TODAY...

_____

_____

_____

## WHAT I'M **LOOKING FORWARD TO** TOMORROW...

_____

_____

_____

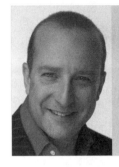

# DAY 19

## Pull yourself out of the stream of judgements

*'Failure is a few errors in judgement, repeated every day.'*

JIM ROHN

If you ever tune into the stream of judgements running through your mind during the course of the day, you could be excused for thinking you were going to drown.

'Oh my god, look at those thighs!'

'Does she really think he's going to look twice at her in that dress?'

'I'm fat. Horrible and fat. Horrible, ugly, miserable and fat.'

The truth is, nearly everyone has a stream of thoughts going on in their head all day long, and if they're not careful, they can start to get stuck inside their own minds.

Today, whenever you meet someone, talk with them or even pass them by in the street, silently say the word 'Peace'. If your brain has been chattering away, it will suddenly go quiet and bring you back into the present moment.

# TODAY'S SUCCESS CHECKLIST

|  | TICK | COMMENTS |
|---|---|---|
| **1** I ate when I was hungry | ☐ | _____ |
| **2** I ate what I *really* wanted | ☐ | _____ |
| **3** I ate consciously | ☐ | _____ |
| **4** I stopped when full | ☐ | _____ |
| **5** I drank water | ☐ | _____ |
| **6** I moved my body | ☐ | _____ |
| **7** I listened to the CD | ☐ | _____ |
| **8** I did the mirror exercise | ☐ | _____ |

## ONE **POSITIVE THING** I NOTICED TODAY...

_____

_____

_____

## WHAT I'M **LOOKING FORWARD TO** TOMORROW...

_____

_____

_____

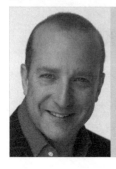

# DAY 20

## What you practise, you become

*'Always act as if you have already achieved what it is you are setting out to accomplish.'*

JOE D. BATTEN

How do you think you'll be different when you've lost the weight you want to lose?

Will you be happier? Have more energy? Feel better about yourself?

While all of these things are possible, they become more likely when you begin to practise them even before you've lost the weight.

Want to be happy, energized and filled with positive self-regard?

Then practise, practise, practise!

# TODAY'S SUCCESS CHECKLIST

|  | TICK | COMMENTS |
|---|---|---|
| **1** I ate when I was hungry | ☐ | _____ |
| **2** I ate what I *really* wanted | ☐ | _____ |
| **3** I ate consciously | ☐ | _____ |
| **4** I stopped when full | ☐ | _____ |
| **5** I drank water | ☐ | _____ |
| **6** I moved my body | ☐ | _____ |
| **7** I listened to the CD | ☐ | _____ |
| **8** I did the mirror exercise | ☐ | _____ |

## ONE **POSITIVE THING** I NOTICED TODAY...

_____

_____

_____

## WHAT I'M **LOOKING FORWARD TO** TOMORROW...

_____

_____

_____

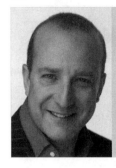

# DAY 21

## See yourself slim

*'Visualization is daydreaming with a purpose.'*

BO BENNETT

Just as athletes rehearse success in their minds over and over again, you need to imagine exactly how you will be when you are thinner. By constantly thinking about how you ultimately want to look, you are programming your mind to make you more and more that way.

Do this simple exercise several times today:

1 Imagine how good you will look when you are a little bit thinner than you are right now.
2 Float into that thinner you. See through their eyes, hear through their ears and feel how good it feels.
3 Now, imagine how good you will look when you are a little bit thinner than that.
4 Once again, float into that thinner you and enjoy the experience.
5 Keep doing this until you can easily imagine being your ideal weight. The more you do it, the easier it becomes.

# TODAY'S SUCCESS CHECKLIST

|   | TICK | COMMENTS |
|---|------|----------|
| **1** I ate when I was hungry | ☐ | _____ |
| **2** I ate what I *really* wanted | ☐ | _____ |
| **3** I ate consciously | ☐ | _____ |
| **4** I stopped when full | ☐ | _____ |
| **5** I drank water | ☐ | _____ |
| **6** I moved my body | ☐ | _____ |
| **7** I listened to the CD | ☐ | _____ |
| **8** I did the mirror exercise | ☐ | _____ |

## ONE **POSITIVE THING** I NOTICED TODAY...

_____

_____

_____

## WHAT I'M **LOOKING FORWARD TO** TOMORROW...

_____

_____

_____

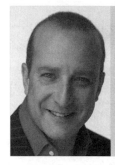

# DAY 22

## Review and renew

*'Learn from yesterday, live for today, hope for tomorrow.'*

ALBERT EINSTEIN

Congratulations!

You are now three weeks into this success journal, and the fact that you are still going means that you really are making changes – inside and out. It's time once again to reflect on how far you've come and refocus on where it is you are heading. Now is an excellent time to compare notes with a buddy and celebrate your success ...

**1** The best things that happened this week were:

**2** My biggest challenges this week were:

**3** I did these things for the first time:

**4** What I learned was:

**5** My top three priorities for the week ahead are:

**a**

**b**

**c**

# TODAY'S SUCCESS CHECKLIST

|  | TICK | COMMENTS |
|---|---|---|
| **1** I ate when I was hungry | ☐ | _____ |
| **2** I ate what I *really* wanted | ☐ | _____ |
| **3** I ate consciously | ☐ | _____ |
| **4** I stopped when full | ☐ | _____ |
| **5** I drank water | ☐ | _____ |
| **6** I moved my body | ☐ | _____ |
| **7** I listened to the CD | ☐ | _____ |
| **8** I did the mirror exercise | ☐ | _____ |

## ONE **POSITIVE THING** I NOTICED TODAY...

_____

_____

_____

## WHAT I'M **LOOKING FORWARD TO** TOMORROW...

_____

_____

_____

# Week 4

# Listen to Your Body!

*'The body never lies.'*

Martha Graham

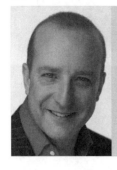

# DAY 23

## Getting to know your body

*'I think awareness is probably the most important thing in becoming a champion.'*

BILLIE JEAN-KING

What's going on with your body right now?

Take a minute now to do a complete inner body scan from head to toe (and yes, that does include 'stomach'!) ... Which parts of your body feel particularly good? Are there any parts of your body that are uncomfortable? Is there any part of your body which is 'unavailable' – i.e. that you can't get a sense of with your eyes closed?

Repeat this exercise at least three times today – make an effort to notice at least one new thing each time. As you become more aware of what's going on with your body throughout the day, it will become easier and easier to stay aware of what's going on with your body while you eat!

# TODAY'S SUCCESS CHECKLIST

| | TICK | COMMENTS |
|---|---|---|
| **1** I ate when I was hungry | ☐ | _____ |
| **2** I ate what I *really* wanted | ☐ | _____ |
| **3** I ate consciously | ☐ | _____ |
| **4** I stopped when full | ☐ | _____ |
| **5** I drank water | ☐ | _____ |
| **6** I moved my body | ☐ | _____ |
| **7** I listened to the CD | ☐ | _____ |
| **8** I did the mirror exercise | ☐ | _____ |

## ONE **POSITIVE THING** I NOTICED TODAY...

_____

_____

_____

## WHAT I'M **LOOKING FORWARD TO** TOMORROW...

_____

_____

_____

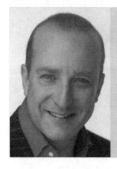

# DAY 24

## Breathe more, eat less

*'The only reason I would take up jogging is so that I could hear heavy breathing again.'*

ERMA BOMBECK

Given that people can go on a hunger strike for 90 days or more without dying, it's probably a bit of an exaggeration to say 'I'm starving' two hours after a Chinese takeaway.

But the body can't survive even five minutes without a healthy supply of oxygen. And when you give the body the oxygen it craves, it will give you more energy and a faster metabolism. Doing this simple breathing exercise before each meal is an excellent way of making sure you're giving your body what it really needs:

1 Breathe in through your nose for a count of five.

2 Hold your breath for a count of twenty. If you can't get to twenty, just hold it as long as you can. Imagine pumping the oxygen through to every cell in your body, giving it the nourishment it truly wants and needs.

3 Now, exhale completely until your body is empty. Stay 'empty' for as long as you can.

4 When your body really wants to breathe in again, let it. Allow your breathing to return to normal.

5 Repeat at least two more times.

# TODAY'S SUCCESS CHECKLIST

|  | TICK | COMMENTS |
|---|---|---|
| **1** I ate when I was hungry | ☐ | _____ |
| **2** I ate what I *really* wanted | ☐ | _____ |
| **3** I ate consciously | ☐ | _____ |
| **4** I stopped when full | ☐ | _____ |
| **5** I drank water | ☐ | _____ |
| **6** I moved my body | ☐ | _____ |
| **7** I listened to the CD | ☐ | _____ |
| **8** I did the mirror exercise | ☐ | _____ |

## ONE **POSITIVE THING** I NOTICED TODAY...

_____

_____

_____

## WHAT I'M **LOOKING FORWARD TO** TOMORROW...

_____

_____

_____

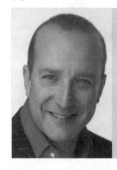

# DAY 25

## Honouring inner wisdom

*'Follow your instincts. That's where true wisdom manifests itself.'*

OPRAH WINFREY

If your body could talk, what would it say to you?

Would it thank you for how lovingly you've been treating it, or would it shrink away like Oliver Twist, afraid to ask you for more?

Throughout the day today, ask your body this question:

'What can I do to take better care of you
in this moment?'

Regardless of whether the answer is 'take a deep breath', 'love me', or 'give me a cream cake!', honour your body's wisdom and do what you can to take care of it.

# TODAY'S SUCCESS CHECKLIST

|   |   | TICK | COMMENTS |
|---|---|------|----------|
| **1** | I ate when I was hungry | ☐ | _____ |
| **2** | I ate what I *really* wanted | ☐ | _____ |
| **3** | I ate consciously | ☐ | _____ |
| **4** | I stopped when full | ☐ | _____ |
| **5** | I drank water | ☐ | _____ |
| **6** | I moved my body | ☐ | _____ |
| **7** | I listened to the CD | ☐ | _____ |
| **8** | I did the mirror exercise | ☐ | _____ |

## ONE **POSITIVE THING** I NOTICED TODAY...

_____

_____

_____

## WHAT I'M **LOOKING FORWARD TO** TOMORROW...

_____

_____

_____

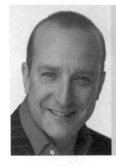

# DAY 26

## Are you thirsty?

*'Water its living strength first shows,*
*When obstacles its course oppose.'*

JOHANN WOLFGANG VON GOETHE

Did you know that when you feel hungry, there is a 75% chance you are actually dehydrated?

This is why one of the most valuable things you can do is to make sure you have a fresh glass of water before sitting down to eat.

One woman who lost 3 stone using my system credited the majority of the weight loss to this one distinction. As she said, 'I had always heard that it was healthy to drink at least eight glasses of water a day, but I could never get myself to do it. By simply drinking a glass of water before eating, I've increased my water intake effortlessly. After doing it for a few weeks, I realized how often I'd been misinterpreting my body's need for water as hunger for food. I now eat much less than I used to, but I never feel like I'm denying myself anything. And when I am hungry, I make sure to eat what I love and love eating it!'

Make a commitment right now to make sure you always have easy access to filtered or distilled water and to drink a glass every time before you eat. You'll be glad you did!

# TODAY'S SUCCESS CHECKLIST

| | TICK | COMMENTS |
|---|---|---|
| **1** I ate when I was hungry | ☐ | _____ |
| **2** I ate what I *really* wanted | ☐ | _____ |
| **3** I ate consciously | ☐ | _____ |
| **4** I stopped when full | ☐ | _____ |
| **5** I drank water | ☐ | _____ |
| **6** I moved my body | ☐ | _____ |
| **7** I listened to the CD | ☐ | _____ |
| **8** I did the mirror exercise | ☐ | _____ |

## ONE **POSITIVE THING** I NOTICED TODAY...

_____

_____

_____

## WHAT I'M **LOOKING FORWARD TO** TOMORROW...

_____

_____

_____

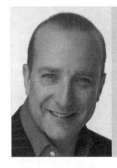

# DAY 27

## Food as fuel

*'Love the moment and the energy of the moment will spread beyond all boundaries.'*

SISTER CORITA KENT

There are two types of energy – potential and kinetic. Petrol is an example of potential energy – in and of itself, it just sits there, but when you stick it in an engine, it becomes 'kinetic' – it fuels the engine to take the car wherever you want to go. As the potential energy becomes kinetic, it gets used up and needs to be replenished.

Similarly, food is potential energy for the engine of your body. This is why it's so important to both eat when you're hungry and move your body.

If you kept driving without putting in enough petrol, what would you expect to happen to your engine? It would continually splutter and stall, and eventually wear out.

On the other hand, if you kept putting petrol into a car without ever driving it, the petrol would begin overflowing everywhere, creating a safety hazard and a bit of a mess.

By balancing eating when you're hungry (filling the tank) and moving your body frequently (driving the car), your body will reward you by taking you wherever you want to go!

# TODAY'S SUCCESS CHECKLIST

|  | TICK | COMMENTS |
|---|---|---|
| **1** I ate when I was hungry | ☐ | _____ |
| **2** I ate what I *really* wanted | ☐ | _____ |
| **3** I ate consciously | ☐ | _____ |
| **4** I stopped when full | ☐ | _____ |
| **5** I drank water | ☐ | _____ |
| **6** I moved my body | ☐ | _____ |
| **7** I listened to the CD | ☐ | _____ |
| **8** I did the mirror exercise | ☐ | _____ |

## ONE **POSITIVE THING** I NOTICED TODAY...

_____

_____

_____

## WHAT I'M **LOOKING FORWARD TO** TOMORROW...

_____

_____

_____

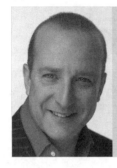

# DAY 28

## The inner smile

*'A smile is a curve that sets everything straight.'*

PHYLLIS DILLER

Here is one of my favourite exercises from *Change Your Life in 7 Days*:

1 Sit comfortably – ultimately you can practise the inner smile anywhere in any position.
2 Allow a smile to dance into your eyes. If you like, raise the corner of your mouth ever so slightly, like someone who knows a really good secret but isn't going to tell.
3 Smile into any part of your body that feels tight or uncomfortable until it begins to ease or relax.
4 Smile into any part of your body that feels especially good. You can increase the smile by expressing gratitude to that part of your body for helping to keep you healthy and strong.
5 Allow the inner smile to reach every nook and cranny of your body.

# TODAY'S SUCCESS CHECKLIST

|  | TICK | COMMENTS |
|---|---|---|
| **1** I ate when I was hungry | ☐ | _____ |
| **2** I ate what I *really* wanted | ☐ | _____ |
| **3** I ate consciously | ☐ | _____ |
| **4** I stopped when full | ☐ | _____ |
| **5** I drank water | ☐ | _____ |
| **6** I moved my body | ☐ | _____ |
| **7** I listened to the CD | ☐ | _____ |
| **8** I did the mirror exercise | ☐ | _____ |

## ONE **POSITIVE THING** I NOTICED TODAY...

_____

_____

_____

## WHAT I'M **LOOKING FORWARD TO** TOMORROW...

_____

_____

_____

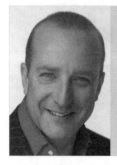

# DAY 29

## Review and renew

*'If you watch how nature deals with adversity, continually renewing itself, you cannot help but learn.'*

BERNIE S. SIEGEL

As you continue changing your eating habits day by day and week by week, it's important to step back from time to time and see how far you've already come.

Take a few moments now to learn from the wisdom of your own experience ...

**1** The best things that happened this week were:

_____

**2** My biggest challenges this week were:

_____

**3** I did these things for the first time:

_____

**4** What I learned was:

_____

**5** My top three priorities for the week ahead are:

   **a** _____

   **b** _____

   **c** _____

# TODAY'S SUCCESS CHECKLIST

| | TICK | COMMENTS |
|---|---|---|
| **1** I ate when I was hungry | ☐ | _____ |
| **2** I ate what I *really* wanted | ☐ | _____ |
| **3** I ate consciously | ☐ | _____ |
| **4** I stopped when full | ☐ | _____ |
| **5** I drank water | ☐ | _____ |
| **6** I moved my body | ☐ | _____ |
| **7** I listened to the CD | ☐ | _____ |
| **8** I did the mirror exercise | ☐ | _____ |

## ONE **POSITIVE THING** I NOTICED TODAY...

_____

_____

_____

## WHAT I'M **LOOKING FORWARD TO** TOMORROW...

_____

_____

_____

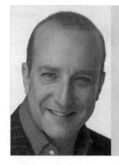

# DAY 30

## Your second check-in ...

*'Success is neither magical nor mysterious.
Success is the natural consequence of consistently
applying the basic fundamentals.'*

JIM ROHN

I have to say I'm impressed. The fact that you've come this far is proof that you have what it takes to change your relationship with food forever. You've probably already begun to notice changes in your energy levels and maybe even your clothes size.

Take some time today to reflect on how things have already begun to change for the better ...

_____

_____

_____

_____

_____

_____

# Michael Gee **LOST 4 STONE**

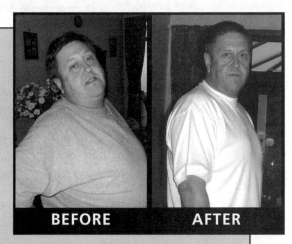

BEFORE AFTER

I had struggled with my weight all my life. About four years ago I was diagnosed with type-2 diabetes, mainly due to being obese, and I was put on medication.

I joined a gym and started swimming five mornings a week, which helped my blood sugar level but had no real impact on my obesity. I heard about Paul's weight-loss programme and attended a seminar in January 2005. By September 2005 I'd lost over 4 stone! It's so easy to lose weight it's immoral.

My family and friends say I look great and ten years younger, but the best thing is that I feel twenty years younger. My GP has reduced my medication and I believe I will soon be off medication altogether. Also, the seminar was a fantastic day. I gained so much that day. I had never enjoyed anything like it and it changed my life forever.

## TODAY I WEIGH

# Week 5

# Keep Going!

*'Motivation is what gets you started.*
*Habit is what keeps you going.'*

JIM RYUN

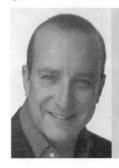

# DAY 31

## Press on!

*'You always pass failure on the way to success.'*

MICKEY ROONEY

As you move into the second month of your 90-day success journal, it's important to keep your passion burning and your commitment alive.

One of my favourite 'power thoughts' on the value of persistence comes from former US president Calvin Coolidge:

*'Nothing in the world can take the place of persistence. Talent will not; nothing is more common than unsuccessful men with talent. Genius will not; unrewarded genius is almost a proverb. Education will not; the world is full of educated derelicts. Persistence and determination alone are omnipotent. The slogan "Press on" has solved and always will solve the problems of the human race.'*

Whether you're feeling excited or daunted as you look ahead, I have only one thing to say to you:

**Press on!**

# TODAY'S SUCCESS CHECKLIST

|   | | TICK | COMMENTS |
|---|---|:---:|---|
| **1** I ate when I was hungry | ☐ | | _____ |
| **2** I ate what I *really* wanted | ☐ | | _____ |
| **3** I ate consciously | ☐ | | _____ |
| **4** I stopped when full | ☐ | | _____ |
| **5** I drank water | ☐ | | _____ |
| **6** I moved my body | ☐ | | _____ |
| **7** I listened to the CD | ☐ | | _____ |
| **8** I did the mirror exercise | ☐ | | _____ |

## ONE **POSITIVE THING** I NOTICED TODAY...

_____

_____

_____

## WHAT I'M **LOOKING FORWARD TO** TOMORROW...

_____

_____

_____

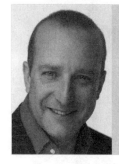

# DAY 32

## The motivation booster!

*'People often say that motivation doesn't last. Well, neither does bathing – that's why we recommend it daily.'*

ZIG ZIGLAR

Here's a simple exercise you can do any time you feel your motivation beginning to flag or your resolve starting to weaken:

1 Make a list of all the reasons you don't want to be over-weight.
2 Make a list of all the reasons you do want to be thin and optimally healthy.
3 Make a list of all the diets you've tried in the past and how long (or short) they lasted.
4 Finally, make a list of the best things you've learned and experienced so far in the process of enjoying eating what you really want when you're actually hungry and stopping when you're full!

# TODAY'S SUCCESS CHECKLIST

|  | TICK | COMMENTS |
|---|---|---|
| **1** I ate when I was hungry | ☐ | _____ |
| **2** I ate what I *really* wanted | ☐ | _____ |
| **3** I ate consciously | ☐ | _____ |
| **4** I stopped when full | ☐ | _____ |
| **5** I drank water | ☐ | _____ |
| **6** I moved my body | ☐ | _____ |
| **7** I listened to the CD | ☐ | _____ |
| **8** I did the mirror exercise | ☐ | _____ |

## ONE **POSITIVE THING** I NOTICED TODAY...

_____

_____

_____

## WHAT I'M **LOOKING FORWARD TO** TOMORROW...

_____

_____

_____

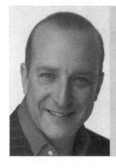

# DAY 33

## Caught in the act

*'Celebrate what you want to see more of.'*

Tom Peters

Ken Blanchard, co-author of the bestselling *One-Minute Manager* books, was at one time a schoolteacher who instituted an unusual practice. Instead of trying to catch students misbehaving or breaking the rules, he would wander around the school seeking to 'catch' kids doing something right.

Today, catch yourself doing as many things 'right' as you possibly can. If you like, go out and buy some gold stars and give yourself one for everything you do well or in keeping with the standards you have set for yourself.

If you really want to make it a great day, catch the people around you doing things right and share your gold stars with them!

# TODAY'S SUCCESS CHECKLIST

| | TICK | COMMENTS |
|---|---|---|
| **1** I ate when I was hungry | ☐ | _____ |
| **2** I ate what I *really* wanted | ☐ | _____ |
| **3** I ate consciously | ☐ | _____ |
| **4** I stopped when full | ☐ | _____ |
| **5** I drank water | ☐ | _____ |
| **6** I moved my body | ☐ | _____ |
| **7** I listened to the CD | ☐ | _____ |
| **8** I did the mirror exercise | ☐ | _____ |

## ONE **POSITIVE THING** I NOTICED TODAY...

_____

_____

_____

## WHAT I'M **LOOKING FORWARD TO** TOMORROW...

_____

_____

_____

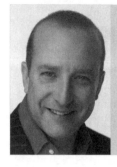

# DAY 34

## Increase the 'fun factor'

*'We don't stop playing because we grow old; we grow old because we stop playing.'*

GEORGE BERNARD SHAW

One of the unsung rules of success is: **What's fun gets done.**

How can you make the process of using this journal and transforming your relationship with food even more fun? Here are some ideas from participants in my seminars:

*Blow up 90 balloons and pop one for each day you successfully complete the programme.*

*Do the programme with a friend – cook great meals for one another, go for walks and share your successes.*

*Keep your eye on the prize – stick a photo of your head on your future body and enjoy the journey!*

Jot down your own ideas here:

*To make this programme even more fun, I could ...*

_____

_____

_____

# TODAY'S SUCCESS CHECKLIST

|   | | TICK | COMMENTS |
|---|---|---|---|
| **1** I ate when I was hungry | ☐ | _____ |
| **2** I ate what I *really* wanted | ☐ | _____ |
| **3** I ate consciously | ☐ | _____ |
| **4** I stopped when full | ☐ | _____ |
| **5** I drank water | ☐ | _____ |
| **6** I moved my body | ☐ | _____ |
| **7** I listened to the CD | ☐ | _____ |
| **8** I did the mirror exercise | ☐ | _____ |

## ONE **POSITIVE THING** I NOTICED TODAY...

_____

_____

_____

## WHAT I'M **LOOKING FORWARD TO** TOMORROW...

_____

_____

_____

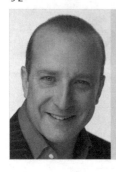

# DAY 35

## Dance!

*'Those who danced were thought to be quite insane by those who could not hear the music.'*

ANGELA MONET

Of all the ways you can move your body, enhance your metabolism and feel great, dancing is probably the most overlooked and most fun.

Today, put some vibrant music on and shake it like you just don't care – if you do this daily, there'll soon be a whole lot less of you to shake!

# TODAY'S SUCCESS CHECKLIST

|  | TICK | COMMENTS |
|---|---|---|
| **1** I ate when I was hungry | ☐ | _____ |
| **2** I ate what I *really* wanted | ☐ | _____ |
| **3** I ate consciously | ☐ | _____ |
| **4** I stopped when full | ☐ | _____ |
| **5** I drank water | ☐ | _____ |
| **6** I moved my body | ☐ | _____ |
| **7** I listened to the CD | ☐ | _____ |
| **8** I did the mirror exercise | ☐ | _____ |

## ONE **POSITIVE THING** I NOTICED TODAY...

_____

_____

_____

## WHAT I'M **LOOKING FORWARD TO** TOMORROW...

_____

_____

_____

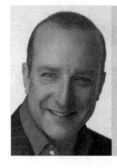

# DAY 36

## The tipping point

*'We first make our habits, then our habits make us.'*

JOHN DRYDEN

There comes a point in the creation of any new habit where it becomes easier to do something than not do it. This is true whether the habit is a negative one (smoking or dieting) or a positive one (exercise, kindness, eating when you're hungry).

With each of the new habits you are creating through doing this programme, notice when you come to 'the tipping point' – that point where it has become easier to eat what you love than what you're supposed to, and when it becomes easier to stop when you're full than to stop when the plate is empty!

# TODAY'S SUCCESS CHECKLIST

|  | TICK | COMMENTS |
|---|---|---|
| **1** I ate when I was hungry | ☐ | _____ |
| **2** I ate what I *really* wanted | ☐ | _____ |
| **3** I ate consciously | ☐ | _____ |
| **4** I stopped when full | ☐ | _____ |
| **5** I drank water | ☐ | _____ |
| **6** I moved my body | ☐ | _____ |
| **7** I listened to the CD | ☐ | _____ |
| **8** I did the mirror exercise | ☐ | _____ |

## ONE **POSITIVE THING** I NOTICED TODAY...

_____

_____

_____

## WHAT I'M **LOOKING FORWARD TO** TOMORROW...

_____

_____

_____

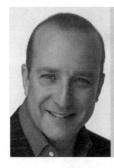

# DAY 37

## Review and renew

*'It's not that some people have willpower and some don't.
It's that some people are ready to change and others are not.'*

JAMES GORDON

You are now more than a third of the way through this 90-day programme. You have set yourself apart from the vast 'herd' of people who say they want to change but are unwilling to do anything to make it happen.

While you celebrate your discipline and perseverance (yes, I'm talking to you!), take some time today to review the week just gone and look forward to the week ahead …

**1** The best things that happened this week were:

**2** My biggest challenges this week were:

**3** I did these things for the first time:

**4** What I learned was:

**5** My top three priorities for the week ahead are:

    **a**

    **b**

    **c**

# TODAY'S SUCCESS CHECKLIST

|   | TICK | COMMENTS |
|---|------|----------|
| **1** I ate when I was hungry | ☐ | _____ |
| **2** I ate what I *really* wanted | ☐ | _____ |
| **3** I ate consciously | ☐ | _____ |
| **4** I stopped when full | ☐ | _____ |
| **5** I drank water | ☐ | _____ |
| **6** I moved my body | ☐ | _____ |
| **7** I listened to the CD | ☐ | _____ |
| **8** I did the mirror exercise | ☐ | _____ |

## ONE **POSITIVE THING** I NOTICED TODAY...

_____

_____

_____

## WHAT I'M **LOOKING FORWARD TO** TOMORROW...

_____

_____

_____

# Week 6

# Emotional Eating

*'It is just about impossible to say grace over a binge.'*

VICTORIA MORAN

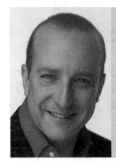

# DAY 38

## Feeling your feelings

*'I think awareness is probably the most important thing
in becoming a champion.'*

BILLIE JEAN-KING

What are you feeling right now?

Instead of going to your head for a verbal answer, take ten seconds or so to scan your physical body from your head down to your stomach. Whatever sensations you notice, I want you to just stay with them for at least 10 seconds …

Have the sensations begun to change?

Every time you allow yourself to feel the feeling sensations in your body instead of cutting off from them or immediately trying to cover them over with food or some other mood-altering substance, those feeling sensations will begin to change.

And when you allow your feeling sensations to flow and change, you will ultimately get to claim the reward of feeling sensational!

# TODAY'S SUCCESS CHECKLIST

|  | TICK | COMMENTS |
|---|---|---|
| **1** I ate when I was hungry | ☐ | _____ |
| **2** I ate what I *really* wanted | ☐ | _____ |
| **3** I ate consciously | ☐ | _____ |
| **4** I stopped when full | ☐ | _____ |
| **5** I drank water | ☐ | _____ |
| **6** I moved my body | ☐ | _____ |
| **7** I listened to the CD | ☐ | _____ |
| **8** I did the mirror exercise | ☐ | _____ |

## ONE **POSITIVE THING** I NOTICED TODAY...

_____

_____

_____

## WHAT I'M **LOOKING FORWARD TO** TOMORROW...

_____

_____

_____

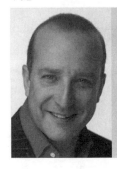

# DAY 39

## Developing your emotional intelligence

*'There is no thinking without feeling and no feeling without thinking.'*

KAREN MCCOWN

All emotions are messages from your unconscious mind. By taking the time to tune into your body and feel your feelings, you are opening up the channels of communication. Here's a simple process from my book *Instant Confidence!* you can use to learn from all your emotions:

1 Clarify the emotion that you are finding uncomfortable. Don't be distracted by thinking about WHY you are feeling it – just focus on the feeling itself. Where in your body do you feel it? Are there certain situations, times, places or people with whom it tends to arise?

2 Next, ask yourself what the feeling is about – what message does it have for you? If you're not sure, it's OK to guess – your guess comes from your intuitive self.

3 Whatever the message, let your unconscious mind know you've received it. If there is any action to be taken, promise yourself you will take it soon – ideally within 24 hours.

4 You'll know you've correctly identified the emotion and its message when the uncomfortable feeling begins to dissolve into the background and your natural, confident sense of ease and well-being returns to the fore.

# TODAY'S SUCCESS CHECKLIST

|  | TICK | COMMENTS |
|---|---|---|
| **1** I ate when I was hungry | ☐ | _____ |
| **2** I ate what I *really* wanted | ☐ | _____ |
| **3** I ate consciously | ☐ | _____ |
| **4** I stopped when full | ☐ | _____ |
| **5** I drank water | ☐ | _____ |
| **6** I moved my body | ☐ | _____ |
| **7** I listened to the CD | ☐ | _____ |
| **8** I did the mirror exercise | ☐ | _____ |

## ONE **POSITIVE THING** I NOTICED TODAY...

_____

_____

_____

## WHAT I'M **LOOKING FORWARD TO** TOMORROW...

_____

_____

_____

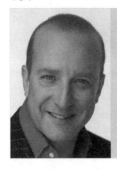

# DAY 40

## What's eating you?

*'There aren't enough cookies in the world to make you feel loved and whole.'*

MICHAEL NEILL

The number one reason people eat when they're not hungry is to fill an emotional hole. But if you're not used to tuning into your body and feeling your feelings, it can be easy to confuse emotional hunger for its physical equivalent.

Here are the two key things to pay attention to:

1 Emotional hunger is sudden and urgent; physical hunger is gradual and patient.
2 Emotional hunger cannot be satisfied with food; physical hunger can.

If you find yourself eating and eating without getting full, you probably don't need more food – you need love.

Throughout the day today, send yourself love at least once an hour and notice the positive difference it makes!

# TODAY'S SUCCESS CHECKLIST

|  | TICK | COMMENTS |
|---|---|---|
| **1** I ate when I was hungry | ☐ | _____ |
| **2** I ate what I *really* wanted | ☐ | _____ |
| **3** I ate consciously | ☐ | _____ |
| **4** I stopped when full | ☐ | _____ |
| **5** I drank water | ☐ | _____ |
| **6** I moved my body | ☐ | _____ |
| **7** I listened to the CD | ☐ | _____ |
| **8** I did the mirror exercise | ☐ | _____ |

## ONE **POSITIVE THING** I NOTICED TODAY...

_____

_____

_____

## WHAT I'M **LOOKING FORWARD TO** TOMORROW...

_____

_____

_____

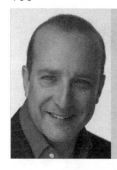

# DAY 41

## The platinum rule

*'Too often we underestimate the power of a touch, a smile, a kind word, a listening ear, an honest compliment, or the smallest act of caring, all of which have the potential to turn a life around.'*

LEO BUSCAGLIA

We are always willing to take more abuse from ourselves than we would ever accept from anyone else. I believe the most important rule when it comes to how you treat yourself is this:

**Do unto yourself as you would have others do unto you.**

If you want to be treated better, begin by treating yourself better.

Do this exercise at least five times today:

1 Ask yourself: 'How can I take better care of myself right now?'
2 Do it!

# TODAY'S SUCCESS CHECKLIST

|  | TICK | COMMENTS |
|---|---|---|
| **1** I ate when I was hungry | ☐ | _____ |
| **2** I ate what I *really* wanted | ☐ | _____ |
| **3** I ate consciously | ☐ | _____ |
| **4** I stopped when full | ☐ | _____ |
| **5** I drank water | ☐ | _____ |
| **6** I moved my body | ☐ | _____ |
| **7** I listened to the CD | ☐ | _____ |
| **8** I did the mirror exercise | ☐ | _____ |

## ONE **POSITIVE THING** I NOTICED TODAY...

_____

_____

_____

## WHAT I'M **LOOKING FORWARD TO** TOMORROW...

_____

_____

_____

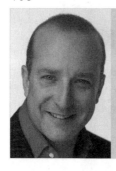

# DAY 42

## Take out your inner critic

*'I must learn to love the fool in me, the one who feels
too much, talks too much, takes too many chances, wins
sometimes and loses often, lacks self-control, loves and hates,
hurts and gets hurt, promises and breaks promises,
laughs and cries.'*

THEODORE ISAAC RUBIN

Here is an exercise from *Change Your Life in 7 Days* that will transform your relationship with your 'inner critic':

1 Stop for a moment and talk to yourself in your critical voice, saying all those nasty things in that unpleasant tone.

2 Now, notice where you make that voice. Does it seem to be coming from inside your head or outside? Is it at the front, the sides or the back?

3 Extend your arm and stick out your thumb.

4 Wherever the critical voice was, move it down your arm to the tip of your thumb, so it's now speaking to you from there.

5 Next slow it down and change the tone of it. Make it sound sexy, or speed it up so it sounds like Mickey Mouse.

# TODAY'S SUCCESS CHECKLIST

|  | TICK | COMMENTS |
|---|---|---|
| **1** I ate when I was hungry | ☐ | _____ |
| **2** I ate what I *really* wanted | ☐ | _____ |
| **3** I ate consciously | ☐ | _____ |
| **4** I stopped when full | ☐ | _____ |
| **5** I drank water | ☐ | _____ |
| **6** I moved my body | ☐ | _____ |
| **7** I listened to the CD | ☐ | _____ |
| **8** I did the mirror exercise | ☐ | _____ |

## ONE **POSITIVE THING** I NOTICED TODAY...

_____

_____

_____

## WHAT I'M **LOOKING FORWARD TO** TOMORROW...

_____

_____

_____

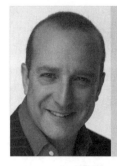

# DAY 43

## The power of appreciation

*'The deepest principal in human nature is the craving to be appreciated.'*

WILLIAM JAMES

Here are some wonderful questions for you to ask and answer throughout the day today:

**1** What's right with my life?

**2** What's working?

**3** Who do I love and who loves me?

**4** What am I most grateful for in my life?

The real value in this exercise is not just the good feelings you will experience in your body but also the changes it will make in your life. By taking the time to deliberately appreciate what you already like and love, you invoke the law of increase:

**You get more of what you focus on!**

# TODAY'S SUCCESS CHECKLIST

| | TICK | COMMENTS |
|---|---|---|
| **1** I ate when I was hungry | ☐ | _____ |
| **2** I ate what I *really* wanted | ☐ | _____ |
| **3** I ate consciously | ☐ | _____ |
| **4** I stopped when full | ☐ | _____ |
| **5** I drank water | ☐ | _____ |
| **6** I moved my body | ☐ | _____ |
| **7** I listened to the CD | ☐ | _____ |
| **8** I did the mirror exercise | ☐ | _____ |

## ONE **POSITIVE THING** I NOTICED TODAY...

_____

_____

_____

## WHAT I'M **LOOKING FORWARD TO** TOMORROW...

_____

_____

_____

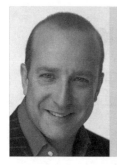

# DAY 44

## Review and renew

*'Sometimes it's the smallest decisions that can change your life forever.'*

KERI RUSSELL

So how are you feeling right now?

Today is an excellent day to reconnect with a supportive friend as you ask and answer the following questions:

**1** The best things that happened this week were:

**2** My biggest challenges this week were:

**3** I did these things for the first time:

**4** What I learned was:

**5** My top three priorities for the week ahead are:

   **a**

   **b**

   **c**

# TODAY'S SUCCESS CHECKLIST

| | TICK | COMMENTS |
|---|---|---|
| **1** I ate when I was hungry | ☐ | _____ |
| **2** I ate what I *really* wanted | ☐ | _____ |
| **3** I ate consciously | ☐ | _____ |
| **4** I stopped when full | ☐ | _____ |
| **5** I drank water | ☐ | _____ |
| **6** I moved my body | ☐ | _____ |
| **7** I listened to the CD | ☐ | _____ |
| **8** I did the mirror exercise | ☐ | _____ |

## ONE **POSITIVE THING** I NOTICED TODAY...

_____

_____

_____

## WHAT I'M **LOOKING FORWARD TO** TOMORROW...

_____

_____

_____

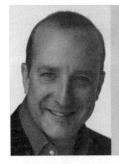

# DAY 45

## Your third check-in ...

*'I eat pretty healthy but I'm not going to not eat a cookie if I want to. I think the more you think about it the more you are going to gain weight – like, 'Oh, I'm depriving myself, so I have to have it!'*

KIRSTEN DUNST

Can you believe it? You're already halfway through the programme! If you're like most people, you're probably feeling one of three ways:

1 Excited about your changing body shape and the additional changes that are happening in your life.
2 Cautiously optimistic – the physical changes haven't been as dramatic as you'd hoped yet, but you can tell that things are definitely different to the way they were before.
3 Stuck, frustrated and contemplating giving up. You haven't lost much weight, and you're beginning to question me, yourself and the programme.

Whichever way you're feeling right now, the most important thing is to keep going. Now that you have a better understanding of what it's like to eat in this new way, you are able to recommit to the programme (and yourself!) at a new level.

*'I, _____, commit to finishing this bloody programme and giving myself a real chance to succeed'*

# Vennice Forbes LOST 4 STONE

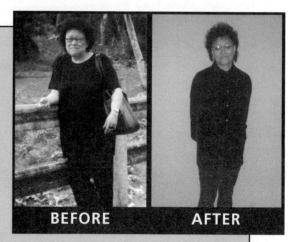

I started using Paul's weight-loss CD about three years ago and lost about 2 stone. However, I still needed to work on my self-esteem and confidence as well as lose more weight, so I attended Paul's weight-loss seminar in February 2005. It was the best thing I ever did.

Bearing in mind it was only a day and there were so many people there, it still boosted the way I felt about myself, reinforcing and building on what I had learned from the CD. I now view food in a totally different way, without the compulsion to comfort-eat and/or overeat. It just goes to show that even at 59 it's never too late to change!

The seminar was incredible and it also introduced me to Paul's NLP courses, which started me on my path to truly loving myself just as I am. I had tried self-improvement/development programmes before, with little long-term success, but straight after my first NLP course my son said he saw huge changes in me, and they did not fade away over time.

# TODAY I WEIGH

# Week 7

# Little Things
# Mean a Lot

*'Confront the difficult when
it is still easy;
accomplish the great task
by a series of small acts.'*

TAO TE CHING

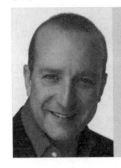

# DAY 46

## Little by little

*'Continual improvement is an unending journey.'*

LLOYD DOBENS

Do little things really mean a lot?

Over the past fifty years, Japanese corporations have gone from strength to strength while many Western companies have struggled to survive. The difference may well be the Japanese practice of Kaizen – a philosophy of continual improvement where small daily actions lead to major lasting changes. To practise Kaizen in your own life, consider the words of John Wooden, one of the most successful basketball coaches in history:

'When you improve a little each day, eventually big things occur. When you improve conditioning a little each day, eventually you have a big improvement in conditioning. Not tomorrow, not the next day, but eventually a big gain is made. Don't look for the big, quick improvement. Seek the small improvement one day at a time. That's the only way it happens – and when it happens, it lasts.'

What are the three smallest changes you could make this week that are liable to make the biggest difference to your ability to follow through with this programme?

Now do them!

# TODAY'S SUCCESS CHECKLIST

|  | TICK | COMMENTS |
|---|---|---|
| **1** I ate when I was hungry | ☐ | _____ |
| **2** I ate what I *really* wanted | ☐ | _____ |
| **3** I ate consciously | ☐ | _____ |
| **4** I stopped when full | ☐ | _____ |
| **5** I drank water | ☐ | _____ |
| **6** I moved my body | ☐ | _____ |
| **7** I listened to the CD | ☐ | _____ |
| **8** I did the mirror exercise | ☐ | _____ |

## ONE **POSITIVE THING** I NOTICED TODAY...

_____

_____

_____

## WHAT I'M **LOOKING FORWARD TO** TOMORROW...

_____

_____

_____

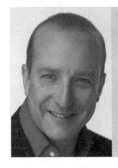

# DAY 47

## Step by step

*'A journey of a thousand miles begins with the first step.'*
LAO TZU

Dr James Hill discovered that there was a difference of only 1,500 to 2,000 steps taken a day between people who were overweight and those who maintained a healthy weight. That may sound like a lot, but it's only the distance of approximately four city blocks. Get creative with at least nine ways you can 'step up' your physical movement today. I've given a suggestion to get you started:

*I can move more today by ...*

**1** *Taking the steps instead of the elevator.*

**2** _____

**3** _____

**4** _____

**5** _____

**6** _____

**7** _____

**8** _____

**9** _____

# TODAY'S SUCCESS CHECKLIST

|  | TICK | COMMENTS |
|---|---|---|
| **1** I ate when I was hungry | ☐ | _____ |
| **2** I ate what I *really* wanted | ☐ | _____ |
| **3** I ate consciously | ☐ | _____ |
| **4** I stopped when full | ☐ | _____ |
| **5** I drank water | ☐ | _____ |
| **6** I moved my body | ☐ | _____ |
| **7** I listened to the CD | ☐ | _____ |
| **8** I did the mirror exercise | ☐ | _____ |

## ONE **POSITIVE THING** I NOTICED TODAY...

_____

_____

_____

## WHAT I'M **LOOKING FORWARD TO** TOMORROW...

_____

_____

_____

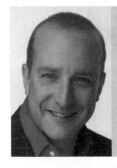

# DAY 48

## Bit by bit

*'If you just keep moving, sooner or later
the finish line will show up.'*

STU MITTLEMAN

Stu Mittleman is the world record holder for the 1,000-mile endurance run and a physical mastery 'guru'. In an interview I once read, a reporter asked Mittleman how he had geared up mentally for running the equivalent of nearly 40 continuous marathons.

Mittleman replied: 'I never ran 1,000 miles – I can't even conceive of running 1,000 miles. All I did was run one mile a thousand times.'

Do you believe you could lose one pound this week by continuing to eat when you're hungry and stopping when you think you're full?

If so, congratulations – you WILL reach your goal!

# TODAY'S SUCCESS CHECKLIST

|   |   | TICK | COMMENTS |
|---|---|------|----------|
| **1** | I ate when I was hungry | ☐ | _____ |
| **2** | I ate what I *really* wanted | ☐ | _____ |
| **3** | I ate consciously | ☐ | _____ |
| **4** | I stopped when full | ☐ | _____ |
| **5** | I drank water | ☐ | _____ |
| **6** | I moved my body | ☐ | _____ |
| **7** | I listened to the CD | ☐ | _____ |
| **8** | I did the mirror exercise | ☐ | _____ |

## ONE **POSITIVE THING** I NOTICED TODAY...

_____

_____

_____

## WHAT I'M **LOOKING FORWARD TO** TOMORROW...

_____

_____

_____

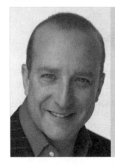

# DAY 49

## One by one

*'You cannot change your destination overnight,*
*but you can change your direction overnight.'*

JIM ROHN

There is a part of your brain called the amygdala whose job it is to keep you safe by preventing you from making major changes in your life. Any time it senses you're going to upset the status quo, it releases stress hormones into your body to 'encourage' you to give up and go back to 'the way things always have been'.

Taking one small action a day outsmarts the amygdala by sneaking past its radar. Yet the cumulative effects of these single daily actions will be nothing short of life-changing. When you are used to doing one thing, two things is easy. When you are used to doing fifty, fifty-one is just as simple.

What is one small daily action you could begin taking to make changes in the important areas of your life?

Here are some examples to get you started ...

To manage stress, I will: *Take one deep breath a day*

To save money, I will: *Put one penny into a jar*

To have more time, I will: *Get up one minute earlier*

Now it's your turn ...

# TODAY'S SUCCESS CHECKLIST

|  | TICK | COMMENTS |
|---|---|---|
| **1** I ate when I was hungry | ☐ | _____ |
| **2** I ate what I *really* wanted | ☐ | _____ |
| **3** I ate consciously | ☐ | _____ |
| **4** I stopped when full | ☐ | _____ |
| **5** I drank water | ☐ | _____ |
| **6** I moved my body | ☐ | _____ |
| **7** I listened to the CD | ☐ | _____ |
| **8** I did the mirror exercise | ☐ | _____ |

## ONE **POSITIVE THING** I NOTICED TODAY...

_____

_____

_____

## WHAT I'M **LOOKING FORWARD TO** TOMORROW...

_____

_____

_____

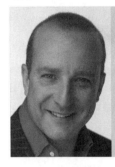

# DAY 50

## Picture by picture

*'All great things have small beginnings.'*
PETER SENGE

Here is a simple way to create a powerful image of yourself being exactly the way you want to be:

1 Imagine a slightly slimmer you sitting or standing in front of you.
2 Now, I'd like you imagine stepping into that slimmer you. See through their eyes, hear through their ears and feel the feelings of your slimmer, more radiant self. And notice that right in front of you is an even slimmer you – sitting or standing a little bit taller, a look of slightly more self-belief behind their eyes, emanating a little bit of extra charisma.
3 Step into this slimmer, more radiant self, and notice that in front of you is an even slimmer self – more self-assured and radiating even more inner beauty.
4 Repeat step three, stepping into slimmer and slimmer versions of yourself until you are looking through the eyes of your naturally slim and radiant self. Be sure to notice how you are using your body – how you are breathing, the expression on your face and the light in your eyes. **Enjoy!**

# TODAY'S SUCCESS CHECKLIST

|   | | TICK | COMMENTS |
|---|---|------|----------|
| **1** I ate when I was hungry | ☐ | | _____ |
| **2** I ate what I *really* wanted | ☐ | | _____ |
| **3** I ate consciously | ☐ | | _____ |
| **4** I stopped when full | ☐ | | _____ |
| **5** I drank water | ☐ | | _____ |
| **6** I moved my body | ☐ | | _____ |
| **7** I listened to the CD | ☐ | | _____ |
| **8** I did the mirror exercise | ☐ | | _____ |

## ONE **POSITIVE THING** I NOTICED TODAY...

_____

_____

_____

## WHAT I'M **LOOKING FORWARD TO** TOMORROW...

_____

_____

_____

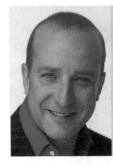

# DAY 51

## Moment by moment

*'Success is how you collect your minutes ... if you don't have all of those zillions of tiny successes, the big ones don't mean anything.'*

Norman Lear

Just for today, collect moments. Perhaps you will see a child hugging its mother and you will experience a moment of unconditional love. Later, a friend will call and you'll have a moment of excitement as you learn something new about a mutual acquaintance. Then you'll be out for a walk and the sun will catch your eye in a certain way that evokes a moment of timelessness.

Normally we walk right by these moments in our lives, distracted by the pursuit of 'more important' things like cooking dinner for the family, finishing the laundry or watching our favourite soap opera.

Today, collect as many of them as you can ...

_____

_____

_____

_____

_____

# TODAY'S SUCCESS CHECKLIST

|   | TICK | COMMENTS |
|---|------|----------|
| **1** I ate when I was hungry | ☐ | _____ |
| **2** I ate what I *really* wanted | ☐ | _____ |
| **3** I ate consciously | ☐ | _____ |
| **4** I stopped when full | ☐ | _____ |
| **5** I drank water | ☐ | _____ |
| **6** I moved my body | ☐ | _____ |
| **7** I listened to the CD | ☐ | _____ |
| **8** I did the mirror exercise | ☐ | _____ |

## ONE **POSITIVE THING** I NOTICED TODAY...

_____

_____

_____

## WHAT I'M **LOOKING FORWARD TO** TOMORROW...

_____

_____

_____

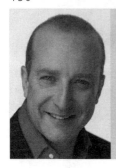

# DAY 52

## Review and renew

*'To God, there is nothing small.'*

MOTHER THERESA

Day by day and week by week, you are becoming the person you have dreamt about for all these years.

Today, take time out to review, renew and celebrate how far you've already come …

**1** The best things that happened this week were:

 

**2** My biggest challenges this week were:

 

**3** I did these things for the first time:

 

**4** What I learned was:

 

**5** My top three priorities for the week ahead are:

   **a**

   **b**

   **c**

# TODAY'S SUCCESS CHECKLIST

| | TICK | COMMENTS |
|---|---|---|
| **1** I ate when I was hungry | ☐ | _____ |
| **2** I ate what I *really* wanted | ☐ | _____ |
| **3** I ate consciously | ☐ | _____ |
| **4** I stopped when full | ☐ | _____ |
| **5** I drank water | ☐ | _____ |
| **6** I moved my body | ☐ | _____ |
| **7** I listened to the CD | ☐ | _____ |
| **8** I did the mirror exercise | ☐ | _____ |

## ONE **POSITIVE THING** I NOTICED TODAY...

_____

_____

_____

## WHAT I'M **LOOKING FORWARD TO** TOMORROW...

_____

_____

_____

# Week 8

# Eating Consciously

*'The secret of health for both mind and body is not to mourn for the past, not to worry about the future and not to anticipate troubles, but to live in the present moment wisely and earnestly.'*

JOHANN WOLFGANG VON GOETHE

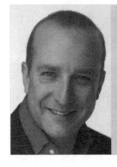

# DAY 53

## The breeze from the refrigerator door

*'Mindfulness can be summed up in two words:*
*pay attention. Once you notice what you're doing,*
*you have the power to change it.'*

MICHELLE BURFORD

Here's a simple way to become more mindful and present in any moment:

- Notice three things you can see.
- Notice three things you can hear.
- Notice three things you can feel.

Practise this throughout the day today, particularly when you are preparing your meals and sitting down to eat.

When you become really present, you may even notice the breeze as you close the refrigerator door!

# TODAY'S SUCCESS CHECKLIST

|  | TICK | COMMENTS |
|---|---|---|
| **1** I ate when I was hungry | ☐ | _____ |
| **2** I ate what I *really* wanted | ☐ | _____ |
| **3** I ate consciously | ☐ | _____ |
| **4** I stopped when full | ☐ | _____ |
| **5** I drank water | ☐ | _____ |
| **6** I moved my body | ☐ | _____ |
| **7** I listened to the CD | ☐ | _____ |
| **8** I did the mirror exercise | ☐ | _____ |

## ONE **POSITIVE THING** I NOTICED TODAY...

_____

_____

_____

## WHAT I'M **LOOKING FORWARD TO** TOMORROW...

_____

_____

_____

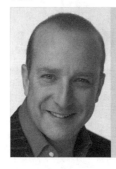

# DAY 54

## Smell yourself slim

*'Nothing is more memorable than a smell. One scent can be unexpected, momentary and fleeting, yet conjure up a childhood summer beside a lake in the mountains; another, a moonlit beach; a third, a family dinner of pot roast and sweet potatoes during a myrtle-mad August in a Midwestern town.'*

DIANE ACKERMAN

According to Dr Richard Bandler, taking a few moments to smell each bite of food before putting it in your mouth alerts your brain to what it is you are about to eat. Your brain then triggers the correct digestive enzymes to be released into both your saliva and your stomach, and whatever you are eating will be digested quickly and efficiently.

Today, take the time to smell each bite of food before you eat it. You'll find it will not only enhance your ability to enjoy each mouthful, you'll feel better afterwards as well.

What do you do if you don't like the smell?

Don't eat it!

# TODAY'S SUCCESS CHECKLIST

|  | TICK | COMMENTS |
|---|---|---|
| **1** I ate when I was hungry | ☐ | _____ |
| **2** I ate what I *really* wanted | ☐ | _____ |
| **3** I ate consciously | ☐ | _____ |
| **4** I stopped when full | ☐ | _____ |
| **5** I drank water | ☐ | _____ |
| **6** I moved my body | ☐ | _____ |
| **7** I listened to the CD | ☐ | _____ |
| **8** I did the mirror exercise | ☐ | _____ |

## ONE **POSITIVE THING** I NOTICED TODAY...

_____

_____

_____

## WHAT I'M **LOOKING FORWARD TO** TOMORROW...

_____

_____

_____

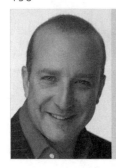

# DAY 55

## Write it down!

*'Tell me what you eat, and I will tell you what you are.'*

ANTHELME BRILLAT-SAVARIN

You have already learned in keeping this journal that there is an incredible value in writing down what you are doing as you are doing it, and in taking the time to review what you have done and to learn from it.

Today, increase your mindfulness of what you put into your body by writing down EVERYTHING you put in your mouth, from the sugar-free breath mint to the evening cup of tea. This is not to make yourself feel guilty about what you are eating – remember, there is no such thing as a forbidden food. It is simply to assist you in becoming more and more aware ...

# TODAY'S SUCCESS CHECKLIST

| | TICK | COMMENTS |
|---|---|---|
| **1** I ate when I was hungry | ☐ | _____ |
| **2** I ate what I *really* wanted | ☐ | _____ |
| **3** I ate consciously | ☐ | _____ |
| **4** I stopped when full | ☐ | _____ |
| **5** I drank water | ☐ | _____ |
| **6** I moved my body | ☐ | _____ |
| **7** I listened to the CD | ☐ | _____ |
| **8** I did the mirror exercise | ☐ | _____ |

## ONE **POSITIVE THING** I NOTICED TODAY...

_____

_____

_____

## WHAT I'M **LOOKING FORWARD TO** TOMORROW...

_____

_____

_____

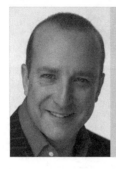

# DAY 56

## Social mindfulness

*'It comes as a great shock to people that they can socialize without shoving food in their mouths.'*

DAVE BARRY

One of the first questions I have learned to ask people who are finding it difficult to lose weight is, 'Are you eating consciously?'

Although they always say 'yes', it often turns out that they habitually eat in social gatherings, chatting away throughout the meal. While it's not impossible to stay conscious and mindful of what you are eating while you are also engaged in conversation, it is bloody difficult.

Just for today, experiment with eating when you eat and socializing when you socialize – you may be surprised at the difference it makes!

# TODAY'S SUCCESS CHECKLIST

|  | TICK | COMMENTS |
|---|---|---|
| **1** I ate when I was hungry | ☐ | _____ |
| **2** I ate what _really_ wanted | ☐ | _____ |
| **3** I ate consciously | ☐ | _____ |
| **4** I stopped when full | ☐ | _____ |
| **5** I drank water | ☐ | _____ |
| **6** I moved my body | ☐ | _____ |
| **7** I listened to the CD | ☐ | _____ |
| **8** I did the mirror exercise | ☐ | _____ |

## ONE **POSITIVE THING** I NOTICED TODAY...

_____

_____

_____

## WHAT I'M **LOOKING FORWARD TO** TOMORROW...

_____

_____

_____

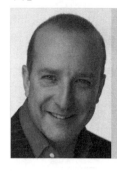

# DAY 57

## Break with routine

*'Fortune and love befriend the bold.'*

OVID

One excellent way to become more conscious of your eating is to change your eating routines. Your conscious mind loves it when you do something the same way every time because it leaves it free to pay attention to something else.

But when it comes to eating, we want to keep our minds front and centre, present and accounted for. What are some of your habitual eating routines?

Do you always eat at a certain time, or in a certain place in the kitchen or sitting room? Do you use the same plates, glasses and cutlery?

Today, change at least one thing from your eating routine. This could be as simple as moving your couch or TV into a slightly different position, or shifting the furniture in your kitchen around. If you're doing it right, it should feel a little bit odd, and maybe even slightly uncomfortable.

As soon as you start getting used to the new way, it's time to break with routine once again!

# TODAY'S SUCCESS CHECKLIST

|  | TICK | COMMENTS |
|---|---|---|
| **1** I ate when I was hungry | ☐ | _____ |
| **2** I ate what I *really* wanted | ☐ | _____ |
| **3** I ate consciously | ☐ | _____ |
| **4** I stopped when full | ☐ | _____ |
| **5** I drank water | ☐ | _____ |
| **6** I moved my body | ☐ | _____ |
| **7** I listened to the CD | ☐ | _____ |
| **8** I did the mirror exercise | ☐ | _____ |

## ONE **POSITIVE THING** I NOTICED TODAY...

_____

_____

_____

## WHAT I'M **LOOKING FORWARD TO** TOMORROW...

_____

_____

_____

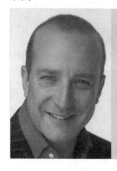

# DAY 58

## Overcoming boredom

*'Life is no brief candle to me. It is a sort of splendid torch which I have got a hold of for the moment, and I want to make it burn as brightly as possible before handing it onto future generations.'*

GEORGE BERNARD SHAW

I have a friend whose young daughter is continually bored. When she can no longer stand to hear her daughter complain, she fixes her a snack.

Allow me to let you in on a little secret:

**The cure for boredom is activity, not food.**

If you find yourself feeling bored today, in search of something to do, move your body. Go for a walk. Dance. Your mind will thank you and your body will be beside itself with joy!

# TODAY'S SUCCESS CHECKLIST

| | TICK | COMMENTS |
|---|---|---|
| **1** I ate when I was hungry | ☐ | _____ |
| **2** I ate what I *really* wanted | ☐ | _____ |
| **3** I ate consciously | ☐ | _____ |
| **4** I stopped when full | ☐ | _____ |
| **5** I drank water | ☐ | _____ |
| **6** I moved my body | ☐ | _____ |
| **7** I listened to the CD | ☐ | _____ |
| **8** I did the mirror exercise | ☐ | _____ |

## ONE **POSITIVE THING** I NOTICED TODAY...

_____

_____

_____

## WHAT I'M **LOOKING FORWARD TO** TOMORROW...

_____

_____

_____

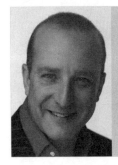

# DAY 59

## Review and renew

*'Reflect upon your present blessings, of which every man has many; not upon your past misfortunes, of which all men have some.'*

CHARLES DICKENS

Did you enjoy your week of eating mindfully? It doesn't have to end today – as you move into the final month of our time together, mindfulness can be a powerful ally as you continue to reprogramme your mind and body to be naturally thin. Take some time today to ask and answer these questions …

1 The best things that happened this week were:

2 My biggest challenges this week were:

3 I did these things for the first time:

4 What I learned was:

5 My top three priorities for the week ahead are:

   a

   b

   c

# TODAY'S SUCCESS CHECKLIST

|  | TICK | COMMENTS |
|---|---|---|
| **1** I ate when I was hungry | ☐ | _____ |
| **2** I ate what I *really* wanted | ☐ | _____ |
| **3** I ate consciously | ☐ | _____ |
| **4** I stopped when full | ☐ | _____ |
| **5** I drank water | ☐ | _____ |
| **6** I moved my body | ☐ | _____ |
| **7** I listened to the CD | ☐ | _____ |
| **8** I did the mirror exercise | ☐ | _____ |

## ONE **POSITIVE THING** I NOTICED TODAY...

_____

_____

_____

## WHAT I'M **LOOKING FORWARD TO** TOMORROW...

_____

_____

_____

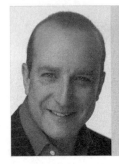

# DAY 60

## Your fourth check-in

*'Never, never, never quit!'*

WINSTON CHURCHILL

How does it feel to be one of the 'few who do' instead of one of the 'many who complain'? You really have set yourself apart by sticking with this programme over the past 60 days, and I'm sure you are very aware of the benefits you are experiencing in your life.

Today, write down at least one thing you've learned about how to take consistent action towards your goals, and the names of at least three people you can share this with.

What I've learned so far from doing this programme:

_____

_____

_____

Three people I can share it with:

1 _____

2 _____

3 _____

# Karen Wheeler **LOST 5½ STONE**

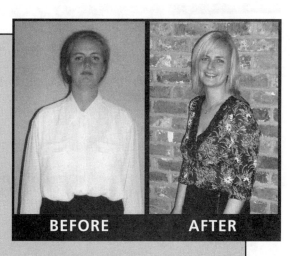

BEFORE  AFTER

Over the last 14 months I have lost over 5 1/2 stone. I never made a point about weighing myself. I would feel my clothes getting looser and then step on the scales and find I'd lost another 7 pounds. Even over Christmas and New Year I lost weight.

When you give yourself permanent permission to eat what you want when you want it, you are no longer concerned about what happens tomorrow. Before, when I dieted, I would have to eat up all the 'bad' foods in the house first! Now there can be chocolate and cake around and it doesn't bother me.

I had been dieting since I was seven years old and nearly 30 years later I finally feel comfortable in my own body. I could look back at the pain and distress of those years but instead I just feel incredibly grateful that I'm on the right path for the rest of my life. Don't waste any more time! Just listen to the CD and look forward to easy weight loss and a relaxed attitude to food.

## TODAY I WEIGH

# Week 9

# Lighten Up!

*'Angels fly because they take themselves lightly.'*

G.K. CHESTERTON

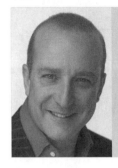

# DAY 61

## Coming out of the closet

*'When I buy cookies I eat just four and throw the rest away. But first I spray them with insect repellent so I won't dig them out of the garbage later. Be careful, though, because that insect repellent really doesn't taste that bad.'*

JANETTE BARBER

What's the craziest thing you've ever done to hide your obsession with food?

Whatever the answer, one of the most powerful things you can do is to go public with it. While I don't normally find myself agreeing with Sigmund Freud, he said one thing I totally agree with:

**Our secrets make us sick.**

Today, 'come out of the closet' about something you've been keeping secret. Make sure you do so with a good friend, and don't be surprised if they try to top you with a 'secret story' of their own!

# TODAY'S SUCCESS CHECKLIST

|  | TICK | COMMENTS |
|---|---|---|
| **1** I ate when I was hungry | ☐ | _____ |
| **2** I ate what I _really_ wanted | ☐ | _____ |
| **3** I ate consciously | ☐ | _____ |
| **4** I stopped when full | ☐ | _____ |
| **5** I drank water | ☐ | _____ |
| **6** I moved my body | ☐ | _____ |
| **7** I listened to the CD | ☐ | _____ |
| **8** I did the mirror exercise | ☐ | _____ |

## ONE **POSITIVE THING** I NOTICED TODAY...

_____

_____

_____

## WHAT I'M **LOOKING FORWARD TO** TOMORROW...

_____

_____

_____

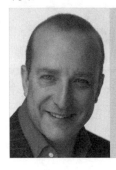

# DAY 62

## The best medicine

*'Laughter has no language, knows no boundaries,
does not discriminate between caste, creed and colour.
It is a powerful emotion and has all the ingredients for
uniting the entire world.'*

DR MADAN KATARIA

According to studies, children laugh up to 400 times a day and adults just 15 times a day. Which to me is proof that there is just too much seriousness in the world!

Madan Kataria MD is known as 'the laughter doctor'. He has founded laughter groups all over the world where people meet to practise 'yogic laughing' for about 15 minutes every day. Yogic laughing is a technique where people are encouraged to laugh for no reason. The reason it is so powerful is that when we pretend to laugh or act happy, our bodies cannot tell the difference between real and pretend and release all the happy positive health chemicals inside us that make us feel good.

So today, whenever it's appropriate (and at least once when it's not!), laugh out loud for as long as you can and kick-start the happy chemicals in your body!

# TODAY'S SUCCESS CHECKLIST

|  | TICK | COMMENTS |
|---|---|---|
| **1** I ate when I was hungry | ☐ | _____ |
| **2** I ate what I *really* wanted | ☐ | _____ |
| **3** I ate consciously | ☐ | _____ |
| **4** I stopped when full | ☐ | _____ |
| **5** I drank water | ☐ | _____ |
| **6** I moved my body | ☐ | _____ |
| **7** I listened to the CD | ☐ | _____ |
| **8** I did the mirror exercise | ☐ | _____ |

## ONE **POSITIVE THING** I NOTICED TODAY...

_____

_____

_____

## WHAT I'M **LOOKING FORWARD TO** TOMORROW...

_____

_____

_____

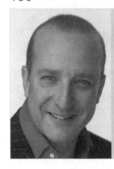

# DAY 63

## Name the game

*'The second day of a diet is always easier than the first.
By the second day, you're off it.'*

JACKIE GLEASON

Every day, we are bombarded with messages telling us not only that we aren't good enough as we are, but that if we will only try this diet or this eating plan, everything will be all right. Today, make note of the many different ways you are invited by television, advertising, stores, newspapers and magazines to ignore what your body wants and eat what the 'experts' tell you is good for you instead.

Here's a list to get you started ...

1 *Fat free*
2 *No sugar added*
3 *Free inside - 10 tips to lose those last 10 pounds!*
4 *As recommended by ...*
5 _____
6 _____
7 _____
8 _____
9 _____
10 _____

# TODAY'S SUCCESS CHECKLIST

|  | TICK | COMMENTS |
|---|---|---|
| **1** I ate when I was hungry | ☐ | _____ |
| **2** I ate what I *really* wanted | ☐ | _____ |
| **3** I ate consciously | ☐ | _____ |
| **4** I stopped when full | ☐ | _____ |
| **5** I drank water | ☐ | _____ |
| **6** I moved my body | ☐ | _____ |
| **7** I listened to the CD | ☐ | _____ |
| **8** I did the mirror exercise | ☐ | _____ |

## ONE **POSITIVE THING** I NOTICED TODAY...

_____

_____

_____

## WHAT I'M **LOOKING FORWARD TO** TOMORROW...

_____

_____

_____

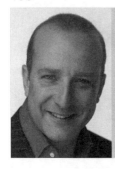

# DAY 64

## A body of light

*'There are two kinds of light – the glow that illuminates and the glare that obscures.'*

JAMES THURBER

An American research study showed that visualizing your body filled with light has a powerful positive effect upon your health and feelings of well-being. Do this now...

1 Imagine that you are preparing your body to bring in more light. What can you do to make your body comfortable and your energy as attractive as possible?

2 Take a deep breath and invite light to come into your body. Imagine it filling your spine and radiating outwards throughout your entire body, until every cell is alive and filled with light.

3 Extend the light out beyond the limits of your physical body. You can imagine it radiating out to fill the room, or gently surrounding you like a cocoon around your body. Keep playing with it until it feels just right to you.

4 Now imagine that you are sending this light to the person or situation that needs it most. Don't worry about running out – the more you share the light, the more your own light is replenished!

# TODAY'S SUCCESS CHECKLIST

|  | TICK | COMMENTS |
|---|---|---|
| **1** I ate when I was hungry | ☐ | _____ |
| **2** I ate what I *really* wanted | ☐ | _____ |
| **3** I ate consciously | ☐ | _____ |
| **4** I stopped when full | ☐ | _____ |
| **5** I drank water | ☐ | _____ |
| **6** I moved my body | ☐ | _____ |
| **7** I listened to the CD | ☐ | _____ |
| **8** I did the mirror exercise | ☐ | _____ |

## ONE **POSITIVE THING** I NOTICED TODAY...

_____

_____

_____

## WHAT I'M **LOOKING FORWARD TO** TOMORROW...

_____

_____

_____

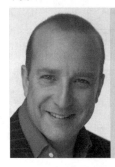

# DAY 65

## Pronoia in action

*'You should view the world as a conspiracy run by a very closely knit group of nearly omnipotent people, and you should think of those people as yourself and your friends.'*

ROBERT ANTON WILSON

I believe there should be a new category of mental health called 'pronoia' – the belief that everything and everyone is conspiring to do you good! Here's a simple way to put your pronoia into action:

Just for today, live as if there is a positive benefit in every one of life's events. Jot down something that happened today and find (or make up!) the positive benefit …

What happened: *I ate about five more biscuits than I intended.*

This is good for me because: *It shows how much I've changed – in the past I would have eaten the whole box!*

What happened:

_____

This is good for me because:

_____

# TODAY'S SUCCESS CHECKLIST

|  | TICK | COMMENTS |
|---|---|---|
| **1** I ate when I was hungry | ☐ | _____ |
| **2** I ate what I *really* wanted | ☐ | _____ |
| **3** I ate consciously | ☐ | _____ |
| **4** I stopped when full | ☐ | _____ |
| **5** I drank water | ☐ | _____ |
| **6** I moved my body | ☐ | _____ |
| **7** I listened to the CD | ☐ | _____ |
| **8** I did the mirror exercise | ☐ | _____ |

## ONE **POSITIVE THING** I NOTICED TODAY...

_____

_____

_____

## WHAT I'M **LOOKING FORWARD TO** TOMORROW...

_____

_____

_____

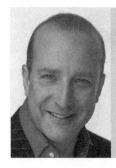

# DAY 66

## The light of the world

*'Let your light shine within you so that it can shine
on someone else.'*

OPRAH WINFREY

One of my absolute favourite quotes in the world comes
from Marianne Williamson, author of the book *A Return to
Love:*

*'Our deepest fear is not that we are inadequate. Our deepest
fear is that we are powerful beyond measure. It is our light, not
our darkness, that most frightens us. We ask ourselves, Who am I
to be brilliant, gorgeous, talented, fabulous? Actually, who are
you not to be?*

*You are a child of God. Your playing small does not serve the
world. There is nothing enlightened about shrinking so that other
people won't feel insecure around you.*

*We are all meant to shine, as children do. We were born to
make manifest the glory of God that is within us. It is not just in
some of us; it is in everyone.*

*And as we let our own light shine, we unconsciously give
other people permission to do the same. As we are liberated from
our own fear, our presence automatically liberates others.'*

# TODAY'S SUCCESS CHECKLIST

| | TICK | COMMENTS |
|---|---|---|
| **1** I ate when I was hungry | ☐ | _____ |
| **2** I ate what I *really* wanted | ☐ | _____ |
| **3** I ate consciously | ☐ | _____ |
| **4** I stopped when full | ☐ | _____ |
| **5** I drank water | ☐ | _____ |
| **6** I moved my body | ☐ | _____ |
| **7** I listened to the CD | ☐ | _____ |
| **8** I did the mirror exercise | ☐ | _____ |

## ONE **POSITIVE THING** I NOTICED TODAY...

_____

_____

_____

## WHAT I'M **LOOKING FORWARD TO** TOMORROW...

_____

_____

_____

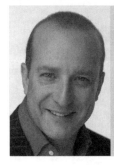

# DAY 67

## Review and renew

*'In the right light, at the right time,
everything is extraordinary.'*

AARON ROSE

By now, you have probably lightened up in more ways than one. As you take the time to review and renew this week, let yourself do so with a light touch and an even lighter heart. Why not invite a friend to join you and share what you've learned?

**1** The best things that happened this week were:

_____

**2** My biggest challenges this week were:

_____

**3** I did these things for the first time:

_____

**4** What I learned was:

_____

**5** My top three priorities for the week ahead are:

   **a** _____

   **b** _____

   **c** _____

# TODAY'S SUCCESS CHECKLIST

| | TICK | COMMENTS |
|---|---|---|
| **1** I ate when I was hungry | ☐ | _____ |
| **2** I ate what I *really* wanted | ☐ | _____ |
| **3** I ate consciously | ☐ | _____ |
| **4** I stopped when full | ☐ | _____ |
| **5** I drank water | ☐ | _____ |
| **6** I moved my body | ☐ | _____ |
| **7** I listened to the CD | ☐ | _____ |
| **8** I did the mirror exercise | ☐ | _____ |

## ONE **POSITIVE THING** I NOTICED TODAY...

_____

_____

_____

## WHAT I'M **LOOKING FORWARD TO** TOMORROW...

_____

_____

_____

# Week 10

# The Weight-Loss Clinic – Your Questions Answered

*'The greatest gift is not being
afraid to question.'*

RUBY DEE

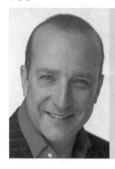

# DAY 68

## Q: Do I have to eat like this for the rest of my life?

That's a bit like asking if you have to enjoy great sex with the person of your dreams for the rest of your life!

- Which bits of the system would you like to change?
- Would you like to stop eating when you're hungry?
- Would you like to stop eating the foods you love and want to eat?
- Would you like to stop enjoying your food as you eat it?
- Would you like to begin making yourself sick from overeating?

Remember, there's nothing in my system designed to punish you or make you wrong – just a recognition that when you are willing to trust your body and stay conscious, your body will reward you with more energy, more aliveness and less wobble.

# TODAY'S SUCCESS CHECKLIST

| | TICK | COMMENTS |
|---|---|---|
| **1** I ate when I was hungry | ☐ | _____ |
| **2** I ate what I *really* wanted | ☐ | _____ |
| **3** I ate consciously | ☐ | _____ |
| **4** I stopped when full | ☐ | _____ |
| **5** I drank water | ☐ | _____ |
| **6** I moved my body | ☐ | _____ |
| **7** I listened to the CD | ☐ | _____ |
| **8** I did the mirror exercise | ☐ | _____ |

## ONE **POSITIVE THING** I NOTICED TODAY...

_____

_____

_____

## WHAT I'M **LOOKING FORWARD TO** TOMORROW...

_____

_____

_____

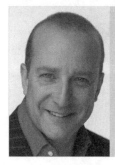

# DAY 69

**Q: It worked great for a month, but then it stopped. Can I come back to it after I try dieting again?**

OK, let's start from the beginning ...

1 Diets are bad for you. They have been proven to lead to significant weight gain over time, they damage your metabolism and sometimes your health, and they reinforce the myth that someone can know more about what your body needs than you do.

2 I have yet to meet anyone who says 'the system stopped working' who doesn't mean 'I stopped using the system'. If you are eating when you are hungry, eating what you really want, enjoying each mouthful and stopping when you think you're full, YOU WILL LOSE WEIGHT or maintain a healthy weight if you're already there.

3 The most common problem I've seen is that after a time, people speed up and begin to go into unconscious eating again. While it's certainly possible to eat quickly and maintain a healthy weight, particularly once your metabolism resets itself, in the meantime, slow your eating down until you are once again completely conscious of each and every mouthful!

# TODAY'S SUCCESS CHECKLIST

|  | TICK | COMMENTS |
|---|---|---|
| **1** I ate when I was hungry | ☐ | _____ |
| **2** I ate what I *really* wanted | ☐ | _____ |
| **3** I ate consciously | ☐ | _____ |
| **4** I stopped when full | ☐ | _____ |
| **5** I drank water | ☐ | _____ |
| **6** I moved my body | ☐ | _____ |
| **7** I listened to the CD | ☐ | _____ |
| **8** I did the mirror exercise | ☐ | _____ |

## ONE **POSITIVE THING** I NOTICED TODAY...

_____

_____

_____

## WHAT I'M **LOOKING FORWARD TO** TOMORROW...

_____

_____

_____

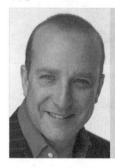

# DAY 70

## Q: Can I 'cheat' and still lose weight?

No, you can't 'cheat' and still lose weight – but not for the reason you think. You can't cheat because there are no foods that you can cheat with. Nothing is forbidden – **nothing**.

Almost all diets agree that there are 'good' foods, 'bad' foods and 'neutral' foods. And, surprisingly perhaps, I agree with them. 'Good' foods are the ones you eat because they taste good, 'bad' foods are the ones you try to convince yourself to eat because they're supposed to be good for you, and neutral foods are the ones you don't eat!

# TODAY'S SUCCESS CHECKLIST

| | TICK | COMMENTS |
|---|---|---|
| **1** I ate when I was hungry | ☐ | _____ |
| **2** I ate what I *really* wanted | ☐ | _____ |
| **3** I ate consciously | ☐ | _____ |
| **4** I stopped when full | ☐ | _____ |
| **5** I drank water | ☐ | _____ |
| **6** I moved my body | ☐ | _____ |
| **7** I listened to the CD | ☐ | _____ |
| **8** I did the mirror exercise | ☐ | _____ |

## ONE **POSITIVE THING** I NOTICED TODAY...

_____

_____

_____

## WHAT I'M **LOOKING FORWARD TO** TOMORROW...

_____

_____

_____

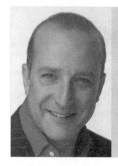

# DAY 71

## Q: How do I eat at a party? I usually don't notice I'm full until it's too late!

Many people feel nervous at parties and then use food and alcohol to try and control their feelings. But the trick to enjoying a party isn't to eat or drink more – it's to place your attention outside of yourself on the people around you. This is the exact opposite of what you have been learning in this book – to eat with your attention on your food and your body.

This is why when you are first learning my system, I recommend avoiding any situation that you know will throw you back into your old habitual eating habits for at least the first two weeks. This gives you time to re-sensitize yourself to your body's hunger and satiation signals.

Once you've grounded yourself in this new way of eating, you can reintroduce yourself to what used to be difficult situations.

If you still find yourself wanting to change the way you feel at a party, you can always use the tapping exercise (see Craving Buster No. 1 on page 220).

# TODAY'S SUCCESS CHECKLIST

| | TICK | COMMENTS |
|---|---|---|
| **1** I ate when I was hungry | ☐ | _____ |
| **2** I ate what I *really* wanted | ☐ | _____ |
| **3** I ate consciously | ☐ | _____ |
| **4** I stopped when full | ☐ | _____ |
| **5** I drank water | ☐ | _____ |
| **6** I moved my body | ☐ | _____ |
| **7** I listened to the CD | ☐ | _____ |
| **8** I did the mirror exercise | ☐ | _____ |

## ONE **POSITIVE THING** I NOTICED TODAY...

_____

_____

_____

## WHAT I'M **LOOKING FORWARD TO** TOMORROW...

_____

_____

_____

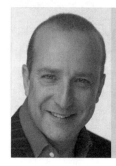

# DAY 72

**Q: I want to eat pasta constantly – is that what my body wants or is it a craving?**

The simplest test for a craving is this:

**If you can't not eat it, it's a craving.**

Fortunately, once you recognize it for what it is, it's the easiest thing in the world to tap it away using Craving Buster No. 1 (see page 220).

Ultimately, the way to eliminate a craving forever is to use Craving Buster No. 2 on page 222 – but be careful! Don't use this unless you're ready to give up eating a particular food forever …

# TODAY'S SUCCESS CHECKLIST

|  | TICK | COMMENTS |
|---|---|---|
| **1** I ate when I was hungry | ☐ | _____ |
| **2** I ate what I *really* wanted | ☐ | _____ |
| **3** I ate consciously | ☐ | _____ |
| **4** I stopped when full | ☐ | _____ |
| **5** I drank water | ☐ | _____ |
| **6** I moved my body | ☐ | _____ |
| **7** I listened to the CD | ☐ | _____ |
| **8** I did the mirror exercise | ☐ | _____ |

## ONE **POSITIVE THING** I NOTICED TODAY...

_____

_____

_____

## WHAT I'M **LOOKING FORWARD TO** TOMORROW...

_____

_____

_____

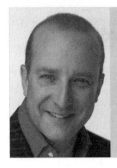

# DAY 73

**Q: After I finish the 90-day programme, can I go back to weighing myself daily?**

By weighing yourself daily, you're just guaranteeing yourself frustration – up one day and down the next. In fact, your weight can fluctuate up to five pounds every single day regardless of how much or how little you eat.

In any case, I believe your weight is the least important measurement of progress you can make. Try these on for size instead:

1 How comfortable do your clothes feel on you?
2 How comfortable do you feel in yourself?

As long as you're feeling better and your clothes are feeling looser, you're making progress!

# TODAY'S SUCCESS CHECKLIST

|  | TICK | COMMENTS |
|---|---|---|
| **1** I ate when I was hungry | ☐ | _____ |
| **2** I ate what I *really* wanted | ☐ | _____ |
| **3** I ate consciously | ☐ | _____ |
| **4** I stopped when full | ☐ | _____ |
| **5** I drank water | ☐ | _____ |
| **6** I moved my body | ☐ | _____ |
| **7** I listened to the CD | ☐ | _____ |
| **8** I did the mirror exercise | ☐ | _____ |

## ONE **POSITIVE THING** I NOTICED TODAY...

_____

_____

_____

## WHAT I'M **LOOKING FORWARD TO** TOMORROW...

_____

_____

_____

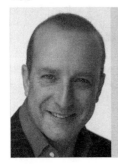

# DAY 74

## Review and renew

*'So long as a person is capable of self-renewal,*
*they are a living being.'*

HENRI FRÉDÉRIC AMIEL

Hopefully, you've already realized that the best answers to your questions are the ones you give yourself.

Today, give yourself the gift of going through the review process in more detail than you normally do – you may be surprised by what you discover!

**1** The best things that happened this week were:

_____

**2** My biggest challenges this week were:

_____

**3** I did these things for the first time:

_____

**4** What I learned was:

_____

**5** My top three priorities for the week ahead are:

   **a** _____

   **b** _____

   **c** _____

# TODAY'S SUCCESS CHECKLIST

| | TICK | COMMENTS |
|---|---|---|
| **1** I ate when I was hungry | ☐ | _____ |
| **2** I ate what I *really* wanted | ☐ | _____ |
| **3** I ate consciously | ☐ | _____ |
| **4** I stopped when full | ☐ | _____ |
| **5** I drank water | ☐ | _____ |
| **6** I moved my body | ☐ | _____ |
| **7** I listened to the CD | ☐ | _____ |
| **8** I did the mirror exercise | ☐ | _____ |

## ONE **POSITIVE THING** I NOTICED TODAY...

_____

_____

_____

## WHAT I'M **LOOKING FORWARD TO** TOMORROW...

_____

_____

_____

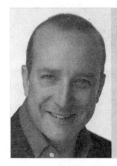

# DAY 75

## Your fifth check-in

*'The first and worst of all frauds is to cheat oneself.'*

PEARL BAILEY

As you reflect back over the past weeks and months, you can no doubt point to one or two key moments when you made a breakthrough decision or did something for the first time that let you know you really have changed.

Take some time today to acknowledge those moments, and in particular to acknowledge yourself for everything you've done to change your life for the better ...

**My 'breakthrough' moments:**

*What happened*            *What changed*

**1** _____     _____

**2** _____     _____

**3** _____     _____

# Beverley Darlison **LOST 4 STONE**

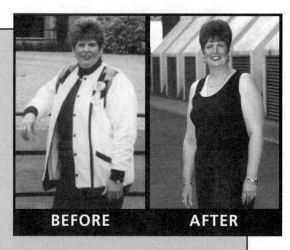

**BEFORE**      **AFTER**

I started dieting at 15 and tried every diet and slimming club going, not once but sometimes four or five times. While I had some initial success at losing weight, it always returned and I ended up gaining more.

I reached my lowest ebb in March 2004 when my health became a real issue. That's when I read Paul McKenna's I Can Make You Thin. This book had to be written about me! I was so inspired I joined Paul's weight-loss seminar. By lunchtime on the day I did not want to eat chips (after Paul's Craving Buster exercise) and for the first time in my life I had to leave some food on my plate. Within three weeks I had lost a stone and had my most enjoyable eating experiences in 33 years. Within five months I had lost 3 stone and was still losing. I have now lost 4 stone.

It has not only changed my appearance but my whole attitude towards life itself. I always felt I was a confident person, but now I know what that really means. Life has become so much more enjoyable for me and all my family and friends – it can for you too.

## TODAY I WEIGH

# Week 11

# Into the Home Stretch

*'Victory belongs to the most persevering.'*

NAPOLEON

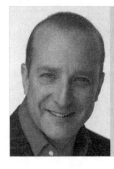

# DAY 76

## Finish what you started

*'Winning isn't always finishing first.*
*Sometimes winning is just finishing.'*

MANUEL DIOTTE

What do you need to do to feel you gave your all to this programme?

As we come into the final two weeks of our time together, I hope you'll consider what it would take to make sure that whatever the outcome, you feel great about your part in making this 90-day journal a true success.

Today, renew your commitment to living each of the four golden rules to permanent weight loss:

1 Eat when you're hungry.
2 Eat what you really want, not what you think you 'should' have.
3 Eat consciously – enjoy each mouthful.
4 Stop when you think that you're full.

**Make the next two weeks your best ones yet!**

# TODAY'S SUCCESS CHECKLIST

|  | TICK | COMMENTS |
|---|---|---|
| **1** I ate when I was hungry | ☐ | _____ |
| **2** I ate what I *really* wanted | ☐ | _____ |
| **3** I ate consciously | ☐ | _____ |
| **4** I stopped when full | ☐ | _____ |
| **5** I drank water | ☐ | _____ |
| **6** I moved my body | ☐ | _____ |
| **7** I listened to the CD | ☐ | _____ |
| **8** I did the mirror exercise | ☐ | _____ |

## ONE **POSITIVE THING** I NOTICED TODAY...

_____

_____

_____

## WHAT I'M **LOOKING FORWARD TO** TOMORROW...

_____

_____

_____

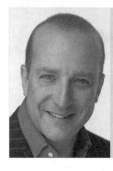

# DAY 77

## Clearing the way

*'It's not that I'm so smart – it's just that
I stay with problems longer.'*

ALBERT EINSTEIN

In 1908, during the aftermath of the Russo-Japanese war which saw more Japanese ships sunk by floating mines than by any other offensive weapon, the British Royal Navy began developing gunboats, fishing trawlers and even private fishing boats into what became known as 'mine sweepers' – specially outfitted ships which could move slowly through enemy waters to locate and destroy mines that had been left behind. Once the mines were cleared, supply ships and additional troops could then be passed through the cleared area to carry out their mission at a much faster rate.

Why the impromptu history lesson?

Because many of the problems you might face over the next few months are predictable, and therefore avoidable.

Take some time today to look around your life for 'pre-problems' – those things which, if you don't take action on them soon, are liable to become a problem two or three steps further down the line. When you find a pre-problem, take action today to prevent it from becoming a 'real' problem in the future!

# TODAY'S SUCCESS CHECKLIST

|   | TICK | COMMENTS |
|---|------|----------|
| **1** I ate when I was hungry | ☐ | _____ |
| **2** I ate what I *really* wanted | ☐ | _____ |
| **3** I ate consciously | ☐ | _____ |
| **4** I stopped when full | ☐ | _____ |
| **5** I drank water | ☐ | _____ |
| **6** I moved my body | ☐ | _____ |
| **7** I listened to the CD | ☐ | _____ |
| **8** I did the mirror exercise | ☐ | _____ |

## ONE **POSITIVE THING** I NOTICED TODAY...

_____

_____

_____

## WHAT I'M **LOOKING FORWARD TO** TOMORROW...

_____

_____

_____

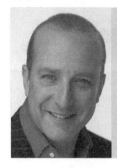

# DAY 78

## Self-intimacy

*'My friends tell me I have an intimacy problem. But they don't really know me.'*

GARRY SHANDLING

One of the 'hidden' benefits of working through this programme is that you've probably been learning more about yourself than ever before.

And that kind of self-intimacy is a precious gift.

Today, I'd like you to up your time in the mirror – spend at least ten minutes with yourself and your body. You don't have to 'do' anything – just see what you see, feel what you feel and stay present with yourself and the process throughout.

Write down what you noticed in the space below:

_____

_____

_____

_____

_____

# TODAY'S SUCCESS CHECKLIST

| | TICK | COMMENTS |
|---|---|---|
| **1** I ate when I was hungry | ☐ | _____ |
| **2** I ate what I *really* wanted | ☐ | _____ |
| **3** I ate consciously | ☐ | _____ |
| **4** I stopped when full | ☐ | _____ |
| **5** I drank water | ☐ | _____ |
| **6** I moved my body | ☐ | _____ |
| **7** I listened to the CD | ☐ | _____ |
| **8** I did the mirror exercise | ☐ | _____ |

## ONE **POSITIVE THING** I NOTICED TODAY...

_____

_____

_____

## WHAT I'M **LOOKING FORWARD TO** TOMORROW...

_____

_____

_____

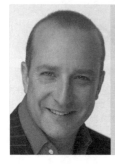

# DAY 79

## A simple recipe (for success)

*'If we are facing in the right direction, all we have to do is keep on walking.'*

BUDDHIST PROVERB

Make a list of what's been moving you towards your goals for this programme and what's been taking you away from them ...

*What's been moving me towards my goals:*

_____

_____

*What been taking me away from my goals:*

_____

_____

Your assignment today is simple – do more of everything on your first list and less of everything on your second!

# TODAY'S SUCCESS CHECKLIST

|  | TICK | COMMENTS |
|---|---|---|
| **1** I ate when I was hungry | ☐ | _____ |
| **2** I ate what I *really* wanted | ☐ | _____ |
| **3** I ate consciously | ☐ | _____ |
| **4** I stopped when full | ☐ | _____ |
| **5** I drank water | ☐ | _____ |
| **6** I moved my body | ☐ | _____ |
| **7** I listened to the CD | ☐ | _____ |
| **8** I did the mirror exercise | ☐ | _____ |

## ONE **POSITIVE THING** I NOTICED TODAY...

_____

_____

_____

## WHAT I'M **LOOKING FORWARD TO** TOMORROW...

_____

_____

_____

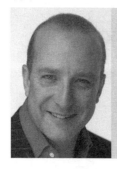

# DAY 80

## Fit for life

*'If it weren't for the fact that the TV set and the refrigerator are so far apart, some of us wouldn't get any exercise at all.'*

JOEY ADAMS

Here is an amazingly simple programme you can use as an aid to fat burning. It will take you about 10 minutes to do, can be done anywhere and needs no special equipment ...

1  For the first minute or so, get your body moving slowly. You can use any form of gentle stretch – it should feel easy and natural, like a cat getting up from an afternoon nap.

2  For the next phase of the programme, aim to do at least five push-ups and five stomach crunches as slowly as possible. See if you can count to 10 on the way up and another 10 on the way down. (If you find regular push-ups are too hard for you, you can begin the push-ups on your knees or even by pushing away against a wall until you become stronger.)

3  For the third and final part of this routine, you can use virtually any activity that causes your body to breathe more deeply and your heart rate to quicken. Walking, dancing, swimming, even climbing stairs will work perfectly well – of course, you can always use a treadmill, stair climber or exercise bike if you prefer. There are only two easy rules to follow – keep moving for a full five minutes, and if the exercise feels too hard, slow down; if it feels too easy, speed up!

# TODAY'S SUCCESS CHECKLIST

| | TICK | COMMENTS |
|---|---|---|
| **1** I ate when I was hungry | ☐ | _____ |
| **2** I ate what I *really* wanted | ☐ | _____ |
| **3** I ate consciously | ☐ | _____ |
| **4** I stopped when full | ☐ | _____ |
| **5** I drank water | ☐ | _____ |
| **6** I moved my body | ☐ | _____ |
| **7** I listened to the CD | ☐ | _____ |
| **8** I did the mirror exercise | ☐ | _____ |

## ONE **POSITIVE THING** I NOTICED TODAY...

_____

_____

_____

## WHAT I'M **LOOKING FORWARD TO** TOMORROW...

_____

_____

_____

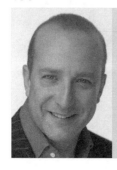

# DAY 81

## Success highlight films

*'The secret of success is constancy of purpose.'*

BENJAMIN DISRAELI

Here is a powerful technique you can use any time you want a boost of confidence, energy and well-being:

1 I'd like you imagine right now that you are watching a movie about a future, more successful you. As the movie plays out on the screen in front of you, you will see many moments of success from your past, and others that have not yet happened. Sit back and enjoy the show!

2 When you're ready, I'd like you to float out of your seat and into that successful you up on the screen. See through their eyes, hear through their ears and feel the feelings of your successful self. Make the colours brighter, the sounds louder and the feelings stronger.

3 Notice where that feeling of success is strongest in your body and give it a colour. Now move that colour up to the top of your head and down to the tip of your toes, doubling the brightness and doubling it again.

4 Float back into your present moment self, being sure to keep as much of the feeling of natural confidence and success as feels truly wonderful.

# TODAY'S SUCCESS CHECKLIST

| | TICK | COMMENTS |
|---|---|---|
| **1** I ate when I was hungry | ☐ | _____ |
| **2** I ate what I *really* wanted | ☐ | _____ |
| **3** I ate consciously | ☐ | _____ |
| **4** I stopped when full | ☐ | _____ |
| **5** I drank water | ☐ | _____ |
| **6** I moved my body | ☐ | _____ |
| **7** I listened to the CD | ☐ | _____ |
| **8** I did the mirror exercise | ☐ | _____ |

## ONE **POSITIVE THING** I NOTICED TODAY...

_____

_____

_____

## WHAT I'M **LOOKING FORWARD TO** TOMORROW...

_____

_____

_____

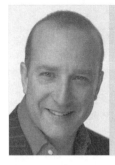

# DAY 82

## Review and renew

*'If a man does his best, what else is there?'*

GENERAL GEORGE S. PATTON

As you prepare for our final week together, take the time to review, renew and celebrate how far you've come. This will allow you to enter into the final week with what Zen monks call 'beginner's mind' – the ability to live each moment as if it is your first ...

**1** The best things that happened this week were:

**2** My biggest challenges this week were:

**3** I did these things for the first time:

**4** What I learned was:

**5** My top three priorities for the week ahead are:

   **a**

   **b**

   **c**

# TODAY'S SUCCESS CHECKLIST

|   | | TICK | COMMENTS |
|---|---|---|---|
| **1** I ate when I was hungry | | ☐ | _____ |
| **2** I ate what I _really_ wanted | | ☐ | _____ |
| **3** I ate consciously | | ☐ | _____ |
| **4** I stopped when full | | ☐ | _____ |
| **5** I drank water | | ☐ | _____ |
| **6** I moved my body | | ☐ | _____ |
| **7** I listened to the CD | | ☐ | _____ |
| **8** I did the mirror exercise | | ☐ | _____ |

## ONE **POSITIVE THING** I NOTICED TODAY...

_____

_____

_____

## WHAT I'M **LOOKING FORWARD TO** TOMORROW...

_____

_____

_____

# Week 12

# A New Beginning

*'Success is not a place at which one arrives,*
*but rather the spirit with which one undertakes*
*and continues the journey.'*

ALEX NOBLE

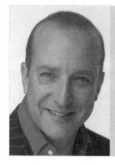

# DAY 83

## There's more to life than being thin!

*'The most important choice you make
is what you choose to make important.'*

MICHAEL NEILL

What would you do if the world was going to end one week from today? In his book *The Power of Full Engagement*, corporate coach Dr James Loehr offers the following questions to help you get in touch with your core values – the most important things in your world:

1 Jump ahead to the end of your life. What are the three most important lessons you have learned and why are they so critical?

2 Think of someone you deeply respect. Describe three qualities in this person that you most admire.

3 Who are you at your best?

4 What one-sentence inscription would you like to see on your tombstone that would capture who you really were in your life?

# TODAY'S SUCCESS CHECKLIST

|   |   | TICK | COMMENTS |
|---|---|---|---|
| 1 | I ate when I was hungry | ☐ | _____ |
| 2 | I ate what I *really* wanted | ☐ | _____ |
| 3 | I ate consciously | ☐ | _____ |
| 4 | I stopped when full | ☐ | _____ |
| 5 | I drank water | ☐ | _____ |
| 6 | I moved my body | ☐ | _____ |
| 7 | I listened to the CD | ☐ | _____ |
| 8 | I did the mirror exercise | ☐ | _____ |

## ONE **POSITIVE THING** I NOTICED TODAY...

_____

_____

_____

## WHAT I'M **LOOKING FORWARD TO** TOMORROW...

_____

_____

_____

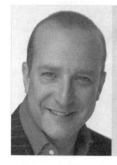

# DAY 84

## A vision for your future

*'Ah but a man's reach should exceed his grasp,*
*or what's a heaven for?'*

ROBERT BROWNING

What is your vision for the future? In other words, how would you like your life to be in five, ten, fifteen or even twenty years from now?

Take some time today to dream. Here are some questions from *Change Your Life in 7 Days* to get you started ...

- If you could be, do or have anything you want, what would you love to be, do and have?
- What would you choose to do if you had unlimited resources?
- What would you love to give back to the world?
- What would you attempt if you knew you could not fail?

# TODAY'S SUCCESS CHECKLIST

| | TICK | COMMENTS |
|---|---|---|
| **1** I ate when I was hungry | ☐ | _____ |
| **2** I ate what I *really* wanted | ☐ | _____ |
| **3** I ate consciously | ☐ | _____ |
| **4** I stopped when full | ☐ | _____ |
| **5** I drank water | ☐ | _____ |
| **6** I moved my body | ☐ | _____ |
| **7** I listened to the CD | ☐ | _____ |
| **8** I did the mirror exercise | ☐ | _____ |

## ONE **POSITIVE THING** I NOTICED TODAY...

_____

_____

_____

## WHAT I'M **LOOKING FORWARD TO** TOMORROW...

_____

_____

_____

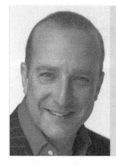

# DAY 85

## Your ideal week

*'Your vision will become clear only when you look into your heart. Who looks outside, dreams. Who looks inside, awakens.'*

CARL JUNG

Today, I want you to review yesterday's questions and write out what an ideal week might be like in your future ...

- How does your week begin?
- How good do you feel?
- Where do you go each day?
- What do you do?
- Who do you spend your time with?
- What lets you know how wonderful your life has become?

On Monday I ...
On Tuesday I ... etc

# TODAY'S SUCCESS CHECKLIST

|  | TICK | COMMENTS |
|---|---|---|
| **1** I ate when I was hungry | ☐ | _____ |
| **2** I ate what I *really* wanted | ☐ | _____ |
| **3** I ate consciously | ☐ | _____ |
| **4** I stopped when full | ☐ | _____ |
| **5** I drank water | ☐ | _____ |
| **6** I moved my body | ☐ | _____ |
| **7** I listened to the CD | ☐ | _____ |
| **8** I did the mirror exercise | ☐ | _____ |

## ONE **POSITIVE THING** I NOTICED TODAY...

_____

_____

_____

## WHAT I'M **LOOKING FORWARD TO** TOMORROW...

_____

_____

_____

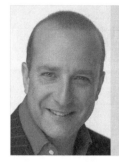

# DAY 86

## Fat is not a feeling

*'It doesn't matter what we do until we accept ourselves.*
*Once we accept ourselves, it doesn't matter what we do.'*

CHARLY HEAVENRICH

Chances are that even after all this time, you may still have days where you hear yourself say, 'I feel fat!' What's important to know is this: **Fat is not a feeling – it's a perception.**

If today is a 'fat day', don't adjust your diet – adjust your attitude. Because if you're 'feeling' fat, chances are there's something else you're not allowing yourself to feel …

1 Tune into your body, particularly the area between your neck and your pelvis.

2 Allow yourself to just be with whatever is going on in your body for at least 30 seconds.

3 When you're ready, let it go. Take at least 30 seconds more to imagine any uncomfortable feelings leaving your body and disappearing into the earth or sky.

4 Now think about someone or something you love and someone or something that loves you. Think about something you're grateful for in your life.

5 When you're feeling more centred and at peace, return to your day refreshed!

# TODAY'S SUCCESS CHECKLIST

|  | TICK | COMMENTS |
|---|---|---|
| **1** I ate when I was hungry | ☐ | _____ |
| **2** I ate what I *really* wanted | ☐ | _____ |
| **3** I ate consciously | ☐ | _____ |
| **4** I stopped when full | ☐ | _____ |
| **5** I drank water | ☐ | _____ |
| **6** I moved my body | ☐ | _____ |
| **7** I listened to the CD | ☐ | _____ |
| **8** I did the mirror exercise | ☐ | _____ |

## ONE **POSITIVE THING** I NOTICED TODAY...

_____

_____

_____

## WHAT I'M **LOOKING FORWARD TO** TOMORROW...

_____

_____

_____

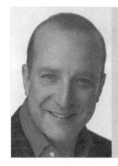

# DAY 87

## Your keys to success

*'Love is the master key which opens the gates to happiness.'*

OLIVER WENDELL HOLMES

A friend of mine was telling me about the moment when he first handed his daughter the keys to the family car and waved a tearful goodbye as she drove down the road on her own for the first time. He knew that for the first time what mattered now was not how much he knew about driving, but how much she had been able to learn.

In a similar way, I have now shared with you the best of what I've learned about how anyone can feel great, lose weight and keep it off for life.

Today, begin to turn my system into your system by writing down your keys to success – the things you have discovered over the past few months which really make the difference between failure and success for YOU ...

*My Keys to Success:*

**1.** ————————————————————————————

**2.** ————————————————————————————

**3.** ————————————————————————————

**4.** ————————————————————————————

**5.** ————————————————————————————

# TODAY'S SUCCESS CHECKLIST

|  | TICK | COMMENTS |
|---|---|---|
| **1** I ate when I was hungry | ☐ | _____ |
| **2** I ate what I *really* wanted | ☐ | _____ |
| **3** I ate consciously | ☐ | _____ |
| **4** I stopped when full | ☐ | _____ |
| **5** I drank water | ☐ | _____ |
| **6** I moved my body | ☐ | _____ |
| **7** I listened to the CD | ☐ | _____ |
| **8** I did the mirror exercise | ☐ | _____ |

## ONE **POSITIVE THING** I NOTICED TODAY...

_____

_____

_____

## WHAT I'M **LOOKING FORWARD TO** TOMORROW...

_____

_____

_____

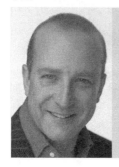

# DAY 88

## What's next?

*'Change starts when someone sees the next step.'*

WILLIAM DRAYTON

The question I am asked most frequently when people have successfully completed one of my programmes is, 'What's next?'

Now that you have successfully taken yourself through this programme, there is one thing you can do which more than any other will help you to build on the momentum you've generated and keep your relationship with eating, food and your body strong:

Volunteer your support for other people who want to lose weight!

Chances are that people have already begun asking you what you're doing differently. Instead of just telling them, you can show them. Take them through the four golden keys. Share the secrets of easy exercise. Encourage them to work through this programme with you as a 'support coach'.

Not only will they thank you, your mastery of the system will grow in leaps and bounds, and you will find it easier and easier to maintain all the gains (and losses!) you have made!

# TODAY'S SUCCESS CHECKLIST

| | TICK | COMMENTS |
|---|---|---|
| **1** I ate when I was hungry | ☐ | _____ |
| **2** I ate what I *really* wanted | ☐ | _____ |
| **3** I ate consciously | ☐ | _____ |
| **4** I stopped when full | ☐ | _____ |
| **5** I drank water | ☐ | _____ |
| **6** I moved my body | ☐ | _____ |
| **7** I listened to the CD | ☐ | _____ |
| **8** I did the mirror exercise | ☐ | _____ |

## ONE **POSITIVE THING** I NOTICED TODAY...

_____

_____

_____

## WHAT I'M **LOOKING FORWARD TO** TOMORROW...

_____

_____

_____

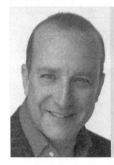

# DAY 89

## Review and renew

*'It's lack of faith that makes people afraid of meeting challenges, and I believe in myself.'*

MUHAMMAD ALI

Did you really believe when you embarked on this journal that you would make it all the way to the end? Whether or not you did, you can certainly believe in yourself now – and you will find that your belief in yourself is one of your most powerful tools for creating lasting changes in your life. Take some time today to once again review the week gone by and to look ahead to the next:

**1** The best things that happened this week were:

**2** My biggest challenges this week were:

**3** I did these things for the first time:

**4** What I learned was:

**5** My top three priorities for the week ahead are:

    **a**

    **b**

    **c**

# TODAY'S SUCCESS CHECKLIST

| | TICK | COMMENTS |
|---|---|---|
| **1** I ate when I was hungry | ☐ | _____ |
| **2** I ate what I *really* wanted | ☐ | _____ |
| **3** I ate consciously | ☐ | _____ |
| **4** I stopped when full | ☐ | _____ |
| **5** I drank water | ☐ | _____ |
| **6** I moved my body | ☐ | _____ |
| **7** I listened to the CD | ☐ | _____ |
| **8** I did the mirror exercise | ☐ | _____ |

## ONE **POSITIVE THING** I NOTICED TODAY...

_____

_____

_____

## WHAT I'M **LOOKING FORWARD TO** TOMORROW...

_____

_____

_____

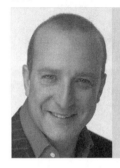

# DAY 90

## Your final check-in

*'So long as a person is capable of self-renewal, they are a living being.'*

HENRI FREDERIC AMIEL

Have you ever seen a performer get a standing ovation? As the applause begins, one or two people stand, then a few more, and soon the whole audience is on its feet, stamping and cheering and applauding out of complete respect for the performer and gratitude for having been able in some small way to be a part of the performance.

I want you to know that if I was there with you now, I would be leading the applause and I would be the very first person to stand! What you have accomplished is phenomenal – and perhaps the best thing of all is that 90 days after you've begun, you don't need me to tell you that any more. You know beyond a shadow of a doubt that what you've achieved is yours to keep forever.

Remember, today's testimonial is the most important one of all – yours! Be sure to get a photo done and paste it into the slot. Write in your story and send it to me c/o Paul McKenna Training, 33 Drayson Mews, London W8 4LY, UK (Attention: Weight Loss Testimonial).

Your Name          **I LOST** _____

| | BEFORE | AFTER |
|---|---|---|
| *Weight* | _____ | _____ |
| *Date* | _____ | _____ |

Perhaps your story will be the one to inspire at least one other person to change their way of eating, change their body and change their life!

Until we meet, please know you have my utmost respect and admiration – it's been an honour to be part of your journey!                    **Paul McKenna**

# Appendix

# The Mirror Exercise

Before you do this exercise for the first time, read through all the steps:

1 Standing in front of a mirror with your eyes closed, recall a specific time when you were paid a compliment by someone you respect or trust. You don't necessarily need to have believed the compliment at the time, but you do need to trust the sincerity of the person who said it. Run through the experience all over again.

2 As you recall the compliment, and the sincerity of the person who said it, pay particular attention to your feelings of trust and regard for this person.

3 When you feel that as strongly as possible, open your eyes, look in the mirror and really see what they saw. Allow yourself to see what someone else has seen and notice how that feels.

4 Finally, imagine taking a picture of yourself just like that. Imagine taking that picture right into your heart. Keep it there so that you can look at it whenever you want to remind yourself how good you can feel.

# Craving Buster No. 1

Before you do this exercise for the first time, read through all the steps:

1   Focus on the food you are craving. Now, rate the craving on a scale from 1 to 10, with 1 being the lowest and 10 the highest. This is important, because in a moment we will see how far you've reduced it.

You must continue to think about your craving throughout the sequence that follows.

2   Take two fingers of either hand and tap about ten times just above one of your eyebrows.

3   Now, tap under the same eye.

4   Tap under your collarbone.

5   Keep thinking about your craving and tap under your armpit.

6   Next, tap on the 'karate chop' point on the side of your hand.

7   Place that hand in front of you and tap on the back of it at the point between the knuckles of your ring finger and your little finger. (Continue tapping that point and thinking about the food you crave throughout steps 8–13.)

8   Close your eyes, then open them.

9   Look down to the right, back to centre, and then down to the left.

10 Rotate your eyes 360 degrees clockwise, then 360 degrees anti-clockwise.
11 Still thinking about your craving and tapping, hum the first few lines of 'Happy Birthday' out loud.
12 Now count out loud from 1 to 5. (1, 2, 3, 4, 5.)
13 Now once again hum the first few lines of 'Happy Birthday' out loud.
14 Repeat steps 2 to 6. Still thinking about what you were craving, tap above the eyebrow, under the eye, under your collarbone, under your armpit and on the karate chop point.

OK, let's stop and check – on a scale from 1 to 10, what number is the craving at now?

If it hasn't completely gone yet, simply go back through the entire sequence again until it does. It may take as many as two or even three times before you have completely eliminated the craving, although most people report getting the craving down to a manageable level on their first or second try. You may even find it has gone completely.

If it ever comes back, you can repeat this process as often as you like, or go through Craving Buster No. 2 overleaf to reprogramme your craving away forever!

# Craving Buster No. 2

Before you do this exercise for the first time, read through all the steps. Remember, only do this technique if you want to stop eating a particular food for good.

1 Think of a food you hate – one that really disgusts you. (A woman on one of my trainings who swore that she loved to eat everything, finally agreed that she found the idea of eating human hair repulsive.)

2 Next, I want you to vividly imagine there is a big plate of the food you hate in front of you. Now imagine smelling and then eating the food you hate, as you squeeze the thumb and little finger of either hand together.

Really imagine the texture of it on your mouth as you squeeze your thumb and little finger together. Imagine the taste of it, squeezing your thumb and little finger together until you feel utterly revolted.

When you are feeling a bit nauseous, stop and relax your fingers.

3 Next, I want you to think of the food that you are going to stop eating. When you think of it, notice that you can imagine what a plate of it looks like.

4 Now, make that picture of the food you like bigger and brighter. Make it bigger still, until it's bigger than you, then make it bigger than that. Continue making it bigger

and bigger and bring it closer and closer and then pass it through you and out the other side. (Most people say that it feels a bit weird to pass the picture through your body – like when a ghost passes through a body in the Harry Potter stories.)

5 Ready? Squeeze your thumb and finger together and remember the taste of the food you hate, while at the same time imagining eating some of the food you like. Now, imagine the food you like is mixed in with the food you hate.

Imagine eating the two foods together, the food you love and the food you hate. Keep imagining the taste and texture of the two together. Keep eating them in your mind, a big plate of them, swallowing them down, as you squeeze your thumb and little finger together. That's it, eat even more, more and more until you can't eat any more, then stop.

6 Think about the food you used to like and notice how it's different now!

You can repeat this process as often as you like until you have completely eliminated your desire for that particular food. You will no longer be a slave to your cravings.